HOT TIPS

1,000 Fashion & Beauty Tricks

BY FRANCES PATIKY STEIN

DESIGNED BY ROCHELLE UDELL

A Perigee Book

Perigee Books
are published by
The Putnam Publishing Group
200 Madison Avenue
New York, New York 10016

Reprinted by arrangement with G. P. Putnam's Sons

Library of Congress Cataloging in Publication Data

Stein, Frances Patiky.
    Hot tips.

    I. Clothing and dress.   2. Beauty, Personal.
I. Udell, Rochelle.   II. Title.
TT507.S76   1983   646   83-8310
ISBN 0-399-50715-9 (pbk.)

First Perigee printing, 1983
Printed in the United States of America
1   2   3   4   5   6   7   8   9

To Mirella

CONTENTS

INTRODUCTION

You have the secret, the key to looking beautiful within reach. You can make it happen! And making it happen is one of the nicest things you'll ever do for yourself . . . it's really very simple.

The three secrets of the most alluring appearance you can have:

1. Looking and feeling your most attractive, *always*

2. Dressing with ease, simplicity

3. Developing and maintaining a consistent, uncomplicated sense of your personal style

The guidelines to follow are all here.

Beauty/Health

Remember: There are no divisions between beauty/health/body/clothes. The root of all is *you*—how you see and feel about yourself totally, from inside to out and back again. How to feel good about yourself, how to look good? The way to begin is with a total body analysis.

Analysis Guidelines

Begin by looking in a three-way mirror—naked—all sides, every detail. Ask yourself:

• Are your legs long or short? Heavy in thigh or calf area?

• Do you have a stomach that is not *flat*? No point in fooling yourself and *trying* to make it disappear. If it's there, it's

there. Fact: you will not always remember to make it "disappear"!

• Are your hips wide?

• Do you have a big derriere, or are you boy-slim?

• Wide waist? Short waist? Long waist?

• Do your shoulders slope down? Are they very wide? Very narrow?

• Big bosom or boy-flat?

• Do you have a short neck? A double-chin problem?

• Is your skin tone rosy and creamy? Sallow? Dark?

• Are you overweight?

Remember that this is an appraisal, *not a condemnation*! You are doing this fact-facing to learn about yourself in order to dress in the manner that best suits you and your body. If you decide to lose weight or begin an exercise program as a result, *Brava*! and so much the better.

Wardrobe Analysis

When planning a foundation wardrobe, think about your needs—how you spend your time and where.

• Do you work?

• Do you entertain much? Where? At home, in restaurants, in a club setting?

• Do you have charity or business meetings and conferences in your life? Lunches? Dinners?

• What are your husband's job's demands on you? Does it include travel to his confer-

ences where you will be with "executive wives"? Lunches? Dinners?

• Do you live in a city where you find yourself in restaurants a lot, or where you go from work to evening without a stop home? Or country, where jeans-dressing can serve you through *days*? Or a suburban town, where you move from city to town and back?

• Do you travel much? For vacations in resort places or for work? To sophisticated cities like Paris, New York, or London? You will want clothes you can pack and unpack easily and that look right anywhere.

• Do you live in a warm, cold, or temperate and changeable climate? (In San Francisco you never pack your sweaters away. In Dallas you need them for the freezing air conditioning. In Miami you rarely ever need more than one or two.)

Ask yourself: In what do I *feel* best? "Best" means most at ease and most attractive. Skirts or trousers? Color? Pale neutrals? Black? The secret to dressing well has to do with finding your personal style and sticking with it like a favorite recipe!

This book is about looking your best. It's the hottest tip of all—everything you need to know about dressing and putting yourself together. And the key is *you!* Your body, your skin, your makeup, your wardrobe, your life, your *style*.

PROPORTION TRICKS

Proportion ideal: A long, slim look. How to get i

RULE: Dark colors slim and elongate. Bright and light colors tend to enlarge . . . they attract the eye.

• To make you look longer, wear a solid color head to toe rather than patterns or prints (or if you must—choose a small, subtly colored, all-over pattern).

• Match or "tone" tops to bottoms: a gray sweater and gray trousers will make you look longer than a navy sweater and gray trousers.

• When wearing skirts, tone stockings to shoes—not to skirt color—this gives the illusion of a longer leg.

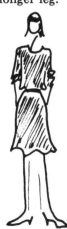

• Wear slim shapes (coats, skirts, etc.) rather than full or broad ones. Avoid big collars, overly wide shoulders; choose narrow rather than wide trousers, etc.)

• Remember: Slim does not mean tight and skinny. It means skimming the body easily without "grabbing." It means a flow of fabric—no constriction anywhere!

• Rule: The thinner the fabric—jersey or soft wool—the more gracefully it falls. Thick tweed is too bulky.

• The darker the tone the more illusion of vertical—no color to distract the eye.

• A tiny bit of shoulder padding gives a lift to your proportion . . . makes you look longer!

• Remember: Lengthening and shortening skirts and tops by even ¼″ can make all the difference in the right proportion for you! Never let anyone say, "Oh, it's so little it's not worth it." It always is.

For the Longest, Slimmest Look, Beginning at the Top To Lengthen Neck

• Keep hair length well off shoulders. Nothing drags the eye down more than hair that is too long!

• Wear open collars on shirts, sweaters . . . The trick—the lower the neckline, the better!

V-neck, oval, or slit-necks—any carved-away to show skin. Avoid turtlenecks, high round crewnecks. Collars that close up high choke you. Avoid anything bulky such as mufflers, scarves, bulky furs, close-to-neck ruffles. If you want the look of a turtleneck, wear a cowl instead. A cowl neck sits away from neck—doesn't cling. And to show even more skin, try pulling one side of the cowl down and holding it off-center with a pin or clip.

If You're Big-Bosomed

• Wear the best support bra possible.

• Wear dark-toned tops—dark tones distract the eye!

• Stay away from tops that are too clingy, complicated, or fussy such as ruffles, breast pockets, etc. The point is to draw attention *away* from the bosom. Always small, "invisible" buttons!

• Avoid double-breasted jackets or coats.

• Never wear wide belts, big collars, necklaces too low.

• Stay away from scarves, mufflers . . . layers that collect just where you don't need bulk!

It has to do with illusion.

• Avoid prints — especially large ones—and *never* horizontal stripes or stitching!

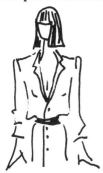

Trick: Wear open-necked sweaters, blouses, dresses. Even the narrowest slit creates a vertical line, and *gives the illusion of a long skinny line.*

If Your Shoulders Slope or Are Too Narrow

Trick: slight shoulder padding in tops. Epaulets and horizontal patterns are great as they give the illusioned width!

• Avoid raglan sleeves—they drag the shoulder line down.

• Breast pockets help; so do lapels on blouses and jackets . . . a horizontal line is what you're after.

If You Are Short-Waisted

Key: Keep tops and bottoms matching or toning *always!*

• Never slice yourself at the waist. Stay away from belts of a contrasting color. Keep belts as narrow as possible and matching the color of the top you are wearing. Trick: Drop belt *slightly* lower than waist to give a *sense* of more torso length.

• A pullover top is best worn *over* skirts or pants, as it keeps waist undefined. Make sure it isn't too long—keep in vicinity of hipbone for maximum elongating effect.

• Never wear wide waistbands; keep them as narrow and as unobtrusive as possible.

Trick: Have your dressmaker or local tailor lower trouser and skirt waists to sit lower on your hips. This gives the *illusion of length.*

If Your Shoulders Are Too Broad

• Remove shoulder pads and epaulets from all garments:

Trick: Have your local tailor adjust set-in sleeve seams by moving them in toward neck by ⅛″. This gives the illusion of a narrower shoulder.

• Raglan sleeves are good. They cut the horizontal line, pull the eye away from the breath of shoulder.

• Avoid all horizontal lines at shoulders: seams, horizontal patterns, yokes, etc.

• Avoid boatneck tops—they are too horizontal a line for you.

Stomach—If You Have One

• Things that cinch you in the middle accent stomach!

Trick: A skirt with gentle gathers at the sides of the front (always keep front smooth!) can help mask stomach. So do side pockets, especially if you use them. It draws the eye away from the bulge. Trouser pleats mask *if* trousers are not worn too tightly. The pleats draw the eye away and create a volume to mask bulge.

Trick: Wear skirts and trousers on the loose side. The fabric doesn't bind and accent stomach this way.

• Keep belts narrow and never tight! and always toned to bottom. This way there is no "slice" in the middle to draw attention to the stomach.

• Stay away from horizontal patterns, big patch pockets, button-front skirts, center pleats (they point to the place you don't want them to point!).

PROPORTION TRICKS

• Wear tops and bottoms toned to one color so that the emphasis is on *one long vertical line* and no attention is drawn to any one spot.

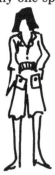

Wide Hips/Big Thighs

• *Never* trouser-pleated skirts or pants! They give a horizontal emphasis where you don't need one.

• *Never* one color on top, another on bottom. Wear pieces of a tone. Keeping one long line means eye is never drawn where you don't want the emphasis—i.e., derriere.

• *Never* clingy fabrics. *Never* horizontal patterns.

• Stay away from too many pleats, gathers, back zippers, back details (stitching, etc.), back pockets (jeans!), big prints! They all attract the eye like arrows.

• Wear gently gathered, narrow soft skirts. Keep them roomy. *The trick is to wear clothes a little on the loose side.* Tight-fitting skirts or dresses cling, bind, and accentuate.

• Stay away from anything bias-cut, as bias means it clings!

• Never wear anything that stops at the waist or just above hips as it becomes an "arrow" to accent hips. Loose tunics, pullovers, or cardigans that cover hips and are toned to skirt or pants are best.

• Never cinch the waist! (An arrow to the widest part.) Stay away from wide belts and contrasting colored belts. They cut your body.

• Check rear views carefully. Make sure skirts and trousers fit well, never ride up, never reveal underpinnings.

• Stay away from skirts and trousers in bulky fabrics as they add weight where you don't need it!

• DARK COLORS ARE SLIMMING; BRIGHT OR PALE ONES ENLARGE.

To Make Legs Look Longer

Remember: The longer your legs look, the slimmer you look. *Your legs can never look too long!*

• Uncuff trousers. No matter how fashionable, cuffs cut the leg.

• Keep skirts no longer than 1½″ below knee. (Find the perfect spot just skimming back of leg where calf begins to curve in.) Skirts that are too long drag—too short and they cut the legs and make them look shorter!

• Ideal: *Create the illusion of one long line.* Wear shoes that are as slim and delicate as possible.

• Always tone stockings to shoe and skirt or pants. You don't want a break in the line.

• 2″ or 3″ heels are pretty—overly high and your calf is accented. (Calf muscles tighten.) You look as though you're on stilts!

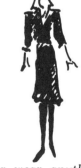

• *Never wear anything that cuts the leg.* No ankle-length pants. No midcalf skirts. No kneesocks. No ankle-strapped shoes. No shoes with bows at instep. No short socks and sandals with skirts. No Bermuda shorts, mini-skirts, etc.

• Avoid skirts and pants that end in any trimming that draws the eye to the leg: no big flowers, edges, no contrasting-colored hems, etc.

• Avoid heavily patterned stockings. *Thin vertical* patterns *toned to shoe and skirt* are best as they draw a long, vertical, leg-lengthening line!

• The slimmer the trouser leg, the better.

Trick: A jacket that stops between the hipbone and the top of the leg-thigh gives the sense of more leg length. Never wear tops and jackets that come too low on thigh. Always match or tone jacket to bottom color!

• Leg lengthener: A front slit skirt, a button-front skirt. They reveal a bit of leg when you walk, give the illusion of length.

Trick: Narrow-lapelled jackets and coats that curve in slightly *above* the waist create a sense of longer legs.

• ⅞ and ¾ coats are great. They make your legs look longer, but only if the skirt that peeks out is the *same tone* as the coat. ⅞ coats are perfect over trousers! That tiny bit shorter coat gives the illusion of long legs. Again, always tone coat and trousers!

If You Are Overweight: Elongaters—Tips on Camouflage Dressing

• Never wear anything too tight. *Never!* Clothes must skim the body so there is a flow of fabric—never any constriction! Thin, soft, graceful fabrics that "move" are best: wool, jersey, thin wool, silk, cotton gabardine. Stay away from stiff, heavy, bulky fabrics (heavy tweeds, terrycloth, thick wool, etc.) They increase the illusion of bulk.

• Wear skirts that fit smoothly over hips and move gently from there (as opposed to waist-full gathers!).

• Wear trousers that sit at the waist and fall plumb-straight to top of shoe . . . slim legs, no cuff.

• *All-of-a-tone!* The more you are one color or tone head to toe, the less the line is broken. The look is long and *slim*.

Slimming Shapes

An easy wrap skirt (never too gathered at waist!)

A lean notched-collared wrap dress in a soft fabric (soft does *not* mean clingy!) The wrap shape gives you skin at neck and leg when you move, thereby creating an elongating center line.

A narrow tunic that falls straight over hips (covering crotch!) over *lean* matching trousers, or a lean matching skirt.

Best coats: A ⅞ coat, raglan-shaped or a cardigan shape (rather than a belted one) to wear over narrow *matching* trousers or a skirt. Make sure coats and jackets are *never* tight and binding across arms, back, bosom, etc.

Any open neckline: A knotched collar, slit-front round-necked top, small cowl on a sweater (rather than a tight turtleneck), narrow lapels.

Best shape: A cardigan jacket that just skims the top of the thigh and a lean matching skirt—ideally a slim wrapped skirt. Think the classic Chanel suit shape and proportion. It's perfect.

Tip: A tiny bit of shoulder padding—as opposed to football ones!—attracts eye up, gives a lift. The magic of a well-placed shoulder pad is that clothes hang with a straighter line and don't collapse on body.

See Maternity section for more tips on overweight and wardrobe suggestions.

BASIC WARDROBE—

- PLAN

This wardrobe is worked out assuming that one wears a balance of trousers and skirts. If you lean more toward one or the other, add one more pair of trousers or one more skirt to starter list. Eliminate one (or all) of the trousers or skirts depending on your preference.

- THIS WARDROBE IS BASED ON PIECES WHICH ARE ALL *TONED TO WORK INTERCHANGE-ABLY*, the theory being that this is the most classic, modern, functional way to dress. It is especially economical. If worked out properly, this way of dressing can make endless looks possible with the greatest *ease* (you should not have to think about it). Through subtle changes, additions and subtractions of accessories this Basic Wardrobe can serve as a foundation for years! REMEMBER: EASE + MOBILITY = MODERN.

The Key: Build a wardrobe as you would a house—foundation first—then add and embellish and enrich season after season, year after year—*always keeping the same foundation.*

- For this you must buy the very *best quality* possible, especially for the foundation pieces. Better fabric = Better Workmanship = Better

Fit = Longest Life. Go for beautiful quality wools, silks, cotton, and linen first.

Remember: Be consistent. *Keep everything toned.* These are the "bones" of your wardrobe, the skeleton. Color-color comes later, when you begin to add pieces!

- How to choose a color family: It is important to know which *tones work best with your skin color* when choosing a color family. Grays look lovely on creamy, *rosy* complexions, but if you tend towards a yellowish or brownish skin cast, the brown/beige family may be better. Navy works well with most skin tones.

- It is equally important to *feel comfortable* and *attractive* in your color family. It must be a *natural* selection.

Test: Look in your closet. What tones do you notice more? If you answer red, then you *really* have to do a rethink! *The classic neutral tones are the key to a skeleton wardrobe—a foundation. They serve as a painter's canvas . . . you embellish upon them!* (You can't do this with red or kelly green as your base!)

Test: Go to a store and choose a crowded rack of expensive trousers or sweaters—all

colors. If you had to put your money on one, which would be your neutral, your *investment*? Some people inevitably reach for black; some, always navy; others, no matter what, always beige!

- The foundation wardrobe is based on solid tones. Have (or choose) a classic color family and stick to it!

The Classic Color Families

- Brown/Beige (including vicuña, taupe to cream . . . all tones from darkest to palest.)

- Black/Gray (including charcoal, taupe [grayed], pale dove to cream, and all tones down from black.)

- Navy (your paler tones can go in either direction: towards grays or beiges . . . . Navy works with both!)

- For a wardrobe with a temperature climate in mind: New York, San Francisco, Chicago, etc. *If a warm climate*, substitute cotton twill or canvas poplin or linen for tweed and gabardine; cotton sweaters and T-shirt jersey for wool sweaters; silky fabrics and thin rayon or cotton jersey for wool jersey. . . . Blouses can also be thin cotton or blends of cotton and rayon, etc. Silk is a major fabric for "late-day"

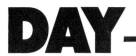

looks! For colors: start with navy, tan, black. Add paler tones. A threesome of off-white or cream trousers, skirt, and jacket—made of linen or cotton poplin—could be the stand-in for the brown/black/cream wool tweed.

Shapes: Classic Is Best

Shapes must be classically simple, pure ... clean! Simple details—nothing overworked —never too "fashiony." If it's *the* newest trendy look, chances are it will *not* serve as a "wardrobe foundation piece." Never dowdy either! *You have to like it a lot to wear it a lot.* THE KEY TO DRESSING AND LOOKING YOUR BEST IS *FEELING FABULOUS*! Dressing must be pleasing or else something is wrong. (See section "What to know about Jackets, Pants, Coats, Skirts" for tips on choosing wardrobe foundation pieces.)

Trick: If one shape suits you and pleases you (a trouser, a blouse, a sweater, etc.) *and* if it works as a good *basic,* don't be afraid to stick to it. Buy several (or *all*) available tones in that shape. Also—as it's rare to find a shape that is perfect, when you do, take advantage of the find!

• If you need a wardrobe which will span season changes, *begin with autumn-winter.* You will be making your major investments here. Winter fabrics are more expensive; therefore clothes are more expensive. You will also have to plan for more pieces with temperature change in mind. You will want to instantly begin looking for *pieces that can span seasons.* *Seasonless* is the word: silk blouses, beautiful wool sweaters (cardigans become summer jackets), raincoats or gabardine coats with button-out linings, jersey pieces, which can be "layered on" in colder weather and work singly in warmer. A beige wool jersey easy skirt from a "cold-weather" two-piece dress can take a cream linen blouse, a pretty belt, and sandals and be turned out for summer travel! Also, warm-weather dressing can be more amusing—more throwaway: a little T-shirt, a cotton gauze skirt and straw shoulder bag are inexpensive and look great! *It's the "big-time investment" clothes (autumn-winter) which take careful selection and savvy planning.*

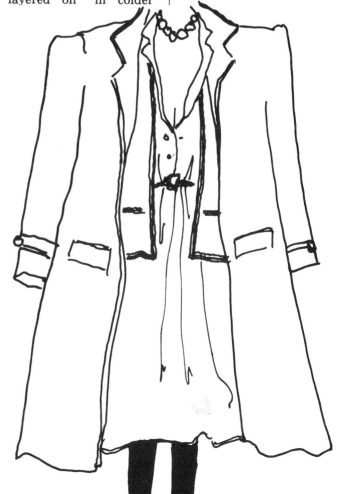

BASIC WARDROBE DAY

Pants
(3)

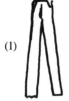 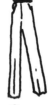 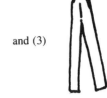 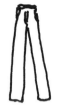

(1) and (2) and (3) (extra) add

choose one (a) Brown Tweed Gray Black (or Navy) Tan
(b) Black/Beige Tweed Flannel Gabardine Gabardine
(c) Navy
(d) Black/Gray Tweed

Jackets
(1)

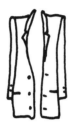 choose one 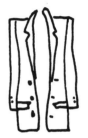 (extra) add
(a) Brown Tweed
(b) Black/Beige Tweed Navy Flannel
(c) Navy or Brown Tweed
(d) Black/Gray Tweed

Skirts
(4)

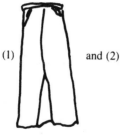 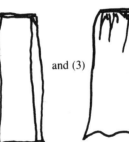 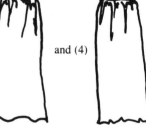

(1) and (2) and (3) and (4)

choose one (a) Brown Tweed Gray Flannel Black or Navy Beige Jersey
(b) Black/Beige Tweed Jersey
(c) Navy
(d) Black/Gray Tweed

Sweaters
Cardigans
(5)

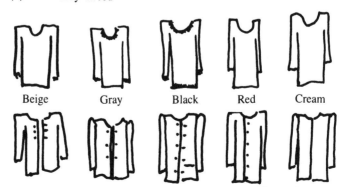

Beige Gray Black Red Cream

Note: Buy crewnecks and cardigans AS SETS when you can.

Blouses

(6)

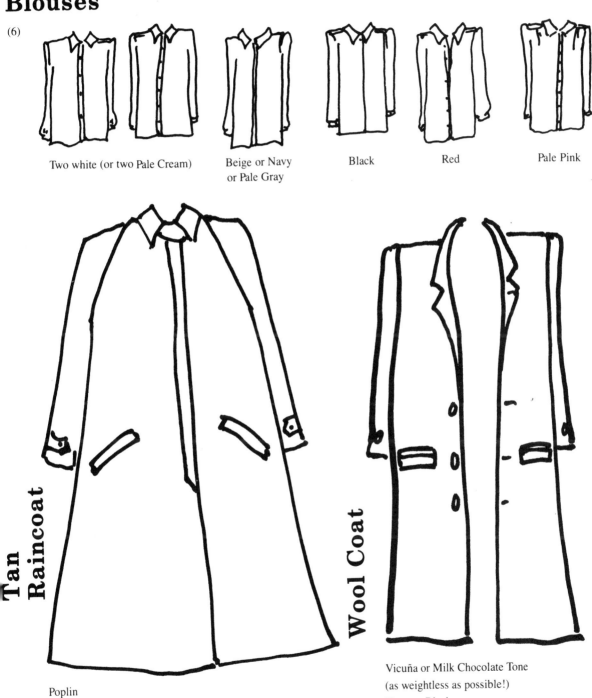

Two white (or two Pale Cream)

Beige or Navy
or Pale Gray

Black

Red

Pale Pink

Tan Raincoat

Poplin
(Button Out Wool Lining Ideal!)

Wool Coat

Vicuña or Milk Chocolate Tone
(as weightless as possible!)
Navy or Black

FORMULAS

How to Use Basic Day Wardrobe— Twenty-six

Note: For clarity we will do "workout" with one color family: brown/beige.

Note: Refer to Belt, Shoe, Jewelry, Handbag, and Scarf Basic Wardrobe Sections for more accessory variations.

1. Brown Tweed Jacket + Brown Tweed Skirt = Suit #1. Add: cream blouse, gold jewelry, brown envelope bag, dark peanut pumps, tan-toned stockings. Perfect for school meetings, office, board meetings, any business or conservative day look! Add: beige cashmere scarf, or if cool, coat in vicuña colored wool.

2. Brown Tweed Jacket + Brown Tweed Skirt = Suit #2. Add: Beige crewneck sweater, pigskin belt, ribbed opaque medium-brown stockings, low-heeled medium-brown moccasins. Add: Brown shoulder bag, carnelian and tortoise shell earrings, carnelian pin in lapel of jacket, one gold, one tortoise shell bangle. Knot a beige cashmere cardigan around shoulders of jacket, tying as you would a scarf or muffler under the collar of jacket. Perfect for office, city day, country charity meetings, etc. A good-looking, easy, pulled-together day look!

3. Brown Tweed Jacket + Gray Flannel Skirt + Gray Cardigan Sweater = Suit #3.

Same accessories as #2—another easy city or business/country look.

4. Brown Tweed Jacket + Brown Tweed Trouser = Trouser Suit. Add: Beige sweater, peanut belt, peanut "trouser shoe" with heel. Tie pale peach silk 36" square scarf at neck. Add: vicuña coat if cold, raincoat or beige cashmere shawl if cool. Add wood and gold jewelry, brown shoulderbag. This is a perfect look for city day or country business day and a great look for travel!

5. Brown Tweed Jacket + Tan Gabardine Pants = City Day Look. Add: cream silk shirt, black wool cardigan over shirt. Belt cardigan closed with brown 1" wide leather belt. Add: brown high-heeled trouser shoe, carnelian-and-wood jewelry, brown leather shoulderbag. To pull it all together, throw a wool blanket-shawl of black-brown-and-beige plaid over one shoulder, for a perfect day city/office turnout.

6. Brown Tweed Jacket + Milk Chocolate Silk Crepe de Chine Shirtdress = Day. Belt dress in peanut leather. Add tan-toned hose, peanut leather pumps, brown shoulderbag. Knot a cream silk crepe de chine scarf in neck. Add gold and wood jewelry: another

great city/work look.

7. Same Jacket and Dress. Add: flat (or low-heeled) moccasins in milk chocolate brown leather with matching opaque stockings. Dress, hose, and shoe are all one tone. Add: beige crewneck sweater *under* dress—wear dress unbuttoned to waist and belted in pigskin. Add gold and tortoise-colored jewelry. Throw jacket over shoulders, and you have a great country/city *easy* dress look!

8. Brown Tweed Jacket + Black Pants (or Skirt) + Black Sweater.
Add: Dark brown heeled moccasin, dark brown bag, gold and wood earrings and bracelets. If skirt, match stocking to shoe.

9. Navy Flannel Jacket + Brown Tweed Trouser + Black Sweater. Add: Shawl + Brown Shoes + Brown Bag + Tortoise-and-Wood Jewelry.

10. Brown Tweed Jacket + Red Sweater + Tan Trousers—same brown shoes and bag.

11. Navy Flannel Jacket + Cream Silk Shirt + Gray Flannel Pants. (The Super Perfect classic look!) Add pigskin accessories, a scarlet wool shawl, and pretty gold jewelry.

Ways (You Will Discover Even More!)

12. Black Crewneck Sweater (cardigan and crew) + Black Skirt = "Dress." Add: vicuña coat, or vicuña-colored wool and cashmere blanket-shawl, or brown tweed jacket; brown-toned stocking and *matching* shoes; brown belt, brown bag, gold and wood jewelry.

13. Beige Jersey Skirt + Beige Crewneck Sweater + Beige Cardigan = "Dress and Jacket" look.
Add: peanut leather accessories, vicuña coat, jewelry—or a big blanket-shawl of beige-vicuña-and-cream plaid.

14. Cream Shirt under Red Sweater + Black Trousers + Brown Shoes and Bag + Black Knitted Shawl = Great city day look! For evening: Brown kid high-heeled *sandals,* sheer sandalfoot stockings to show scarlet toenails, small brown kid bag with a red silk tassel. (Buy tassels in drapery stores and attach to zipper pull of bag!) Add: gold jewelry.

15. Red Cardigan Sweater + Cream Shirt + Gray Flannel Skirt. Add pigskin accessories, matching tan-toned stocking, brown-toned bag, pretty jewelry.

16. Brown Tweed Jacket + Red Blouse + Tan Trousers. Add: peanut kid belt, wood and gold jewelry, peanut trouser shoe.

17. Navy Flannel Jacket + Cream Blouse + Brown Tweed Skirt. Add: brown-toned stockings and shoe, brown belt with gold buckle, gold and wood jewelry.

18. Brown Tweed Jacket + Black Skirt + Black Sweater (or Black Blouse).
Add: dark brown stockings and shoe. Gold jewelry.

19. Black Cardigan + Black Crewneck + Tan Jersey Skirt. Add: pigskin accessories, gold jewelry. For dash—a plaid shawl.

20. Navy Jacket + Black Sweater + Black Pants.
Add: brown leather accessories, gold and wood jewelry for a very chic work look! Throw black shawl over shoulder if cool.

21. Gray Sweater + Gray Skirt + Brown Tweed Jacket (or Vicuña Coat) over shoulders, medium-brown stockings and shoe, plus wood and gold jewelry.

22. Gray Sweater + Gray Trousers + Navy Blazer + Peanut leather accessories.

23. Trick: Black Skirt + Black Sweaters (Crewneck tucked in, Cardigan as Jacket) = *Dress!*

Add: narrow brown and black woven leather belt with gold buckle, gold and carnelian earrings, gold necklaces, pretty brown kid shoes, brown-toned sheer stockings. A perfect turnout! Throw a bordeaux or dark cobalt blue shawl over one shoulder . . . for a great-looking day turnout. Add narrow gold belt, gold earrings, bracelets, bare *black* satin sandals, sheer stockings, and you have an instant-dinner look!

24. Trick: Beige Sweater + Beige Skirt = *Dress!*
Add: peanut leather accessories, gold jewelry (or jade and gold), and for dash, a scarlet blanket shawl. Evening look: brown kid sandals, narrow gold belt, more jewels.

25. Trick: Black Sweater + Black Trousers = Evening!
Add: gold cuffs, gold earrings, scarlet kid sandals, a scarlet thin wool and silk shawl . . . fabulous easy evening!

26. Trick: *Pink* Silk Blouse + Gray Flannel Trousers.
Add: Gold belt, gold sandals, pink quartz-and-gold necklaces, gold cuffs. Pull your hair back and tuck a gardenia into the rubberband—or tuck a gardenia into the buckle of belt—for an extra-easy, instant, and *pretty* evening at-home look.

JACKETS

The Classics

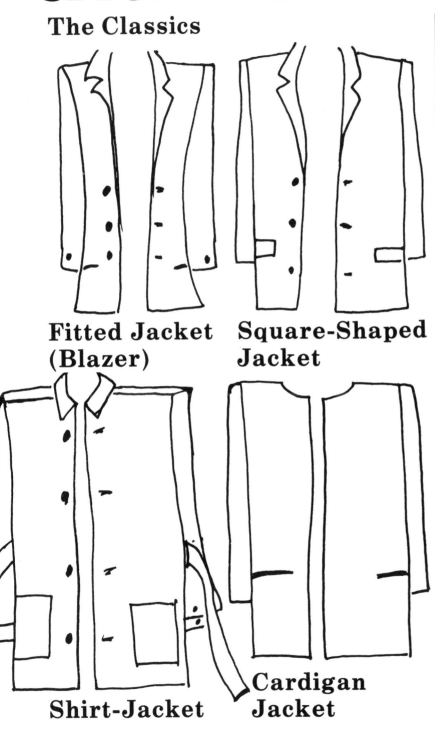

Fitted Jacket (Blazer)

Square-Shaped Jacket

Shirt-Jacket

Cardigan Jacket

• **IDEAL LENGTH:** *Just covering the derriere where legs begin.* This goes especially for *jackets worn over trousers* ... Nothing looks worse (unless you've an extra-perfect body) than a jacket hitting mid-derriere—it's like arrows pointing to the wrong place!

• *Key jacket length for skirts*: (The ideal is to find the perfect jacket length to wear over *both trousers and skirts.* Just covering the derriere is the guideline to use. If jackets worn over skirts are too long, they tend to make one look dumpy. There should always be the sense of *more skirt than jacket* for good balance *and* maximum illusion of a long narrow body! (When you want even more length, tone your stocking and shoe to *color* of skirt.)

• Remember: With jacket lengths, experimenting with as little as ⅛″ of hem can make all the difference between "the perfect length" and *too long* or *too short*! Try the walking test . . . make sure the jacket still covers your behind! We are speaking of fractions of an inch here!

FABRICS: Always remember that classic materials are best. Choose from subtle tweeds, corduroy, flannel (especially navy!), wool and cotton gabardine, linen, cotton twill, velvet to wear day and night, lovely soft suede.

• Watch out for linings. They must be of soft silky material if at all! The most modern jackets are often unlined and nicely finished along seams. Make sure linings don't "fight" the jacket fabric and pull the jacket shape askew.

COLORS: Classic basic colors and tones are best—browns, beiges, navy, grays, black; cream or white for sun places. Remember, you want to be able to move these jackets through your wardrobe, season after season. A hot-violet satin jacket is fun but how many times will you want to look at it, much less wear it!

TRICK: If the jacket comes with matching trousers and/or skirt, buy them. Some designers make several pieces in the same fabric in a collection for just this reason—Collectables! You will instantly have a pulled-together, no-need-to-think-about-it look!

• Remember: Classic jackets— as well as the other basic pieces: pants, coats, skirts— are **investments**. You buy them with a goal: *to wear them often and for a long time.*

• Therefore *buy the best you can afford.* This means good fabric, good workmanship, better fit, and longest life!

• Ideal sleeve length: Test— When you bend hand up, bottom of sleeve should just graze hand.

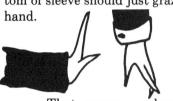

That means a sleeve should just cover the wristbone. *Trick* for making sleeves look longer when you are caught short: Make sure the cuff of your shirt or sweater shows below the sleeve of your jacket. In men's wear language this is called "shooting your cuffs." For a pretty look, try turning your shirt cuff back *over* the jacket cuff. This is particularly nice to do with French-cuffed shirts, the kind that take cufflinks!

The Fitted Jacket (Blazer)

Single- or double-breasted, set-in sleeves, shaped (curved) at waist.
• The first rule for a basic blazer: Single-breasted is best. It is a sparer proportion, easier to handle (less fabric), less bulky, and it moves over most skirts and trousers with equal ease.
Look for:
• Lapels which are not too big or too pointed (or for that matter, too skinny!). The point: classic and conservative. A nice median lapel is around 2½″ wide. It will look "mod-

ern" for the longest time, like a *classic*, conservative man's lapel!

• Simple buttons. Always! For all jackets, coats, blouses—for anything! The best buttons are toned to the color of the fabric. The shape: classic four-hole buttons like the ones on a man's suit. This means that you will be able to wear the jacket both day and evening by changing what's underneath, adding or subtracting accessories without a button clash.

• The shoulders of jacket and collar must *sit* and *balance* on your own shoulders and neck. Test: If the collar grazes your neck when you hold your head straight or slightly raised, or sits so low that it gaps at the back of the neck, there is something out of balance. If you feel a pull across shoulders or a pressure downward on the shoulders, something is wrong. If you can't comfortably move your arms over your head— but instead at mid-chest feel that you are caught in a vise-like grip—all wrong!

• Padding: Shoulders with a bit of padding are great only if it doesn't point up or protrude more than ½″ to ¾″ off your natural shoulder line. Jacket shoulders must always sit on a perfect, arrow-straight horizontal. Jacket sleeves should fall smoothly from the jacket shoulder and never indent under the shoulder pad or shoulder seam.

• Never, ever bust darts in a jacket. It instantly means that the jacket hasn't been tailored with an expert hand.

• The body of the jacket should move smoothly and subtly into the curve at your waist and then out and *down* (see sketch)—not out and out . . . you do not want a flared skirt on your blazer!

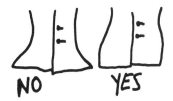

• Check side view. The jacket hem should be *straight*—never dipping in back or in front, never, ever angled so that the back is longer than the front. If you can see the angle it is wrong! If there is one, it should be so subtle it is literally invisible.

• If there is a back vent or back slit in the jacket, the vent should close *straight* and smooth and never, ever gap! Test: Stand straight and have a look in a three-way mirror.

TRICK for more leg length: Look for a blazer that tapers a bit *above* your natural waist (the shape of a riding or hack-

ing jacket) and remember that all in-and-out curves should be subtle—*barely noticeable* is the key! The effect of the *illusion* of a higher waist instantly makes your legs look longer. It has to do with fractions of an inch!

The Square-Shaped Jacket

• This shape is basically a collared version of #4, the Cardigan. It is one of the most body-flattering and easy-to-wear shapes. The key to fit: A square-shaped jacket must fall die-straight from shoulder to hem. Look for ones with small as opposed to oversized collars—no matter if they have notched lapels or short shirt-collars. This will automatically insure a longer wearing life!

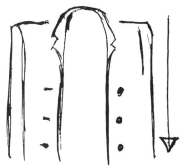

LENGTH: The length of this jacket shape often varies . . . from just grazing the top of hipbone to ¾ (mid-thigh) long. Here is where knowing (a) your wardrobe (Do you own more pants then skirts?) and (b) your body (Do

you have derriere-hip problems?) counts.

• The hipbone to top-of-leg length is great to wear with *skirts* as it gives the *illusion of more leg length*. It must be toned to the skirt and is *never* toned darker than the skirt.

• If you want *leg length, the general rule*: Always keep darker tones on bottom, lighter tones on top.

• If you want to minimize top proportion (wide shoulders, a big bosom, etc.), go for a **shade** *darker* on top, a **tone** *lighter* on bottom, but only if you have the leg length to keep you from looking dumpy! *Match colors exactly*.

• If the jacket length is hipbone to top-of-leg long it is not great for trousers unless you have a *perfect* body. It cuts across mid-derriere at a point where it accents hips and derriere like arrows!

RULE: Make sure that any jacket worn with trousers always covers the derriere, even when you walk. And remember, we are talking about fractions of an inch!

• The longer, mid-thigh, ¾ length is a great length with trousers. It covers hips, thighs, and derriere. Provided it is toned to the trouser color (remembering the length rule: "lighter on top, darker below"), *it is a great body-lengthening proportion!* It can make you look like you have endlessly long legs!

• If you wear both skirts and trousers interchangeably, look for a jacket length that just covers the derriere.

Details:

• Again, never bust darts!

• Watch out for too many pockets. All too often this shape is designed with two breast pockets as well as two hand pockets. Breast pockets attract the eye to the bosom. They are also a neck shortener as they make one look top heavy.

• Generally, the fewer the pockets, the better. The jacket is then more adaptable to accessory changes. This means a longer wearing life!

FIT: Stand sideways. The hem of this jacket has to be perfectly even. Otherwise it is balanced badly and never looks right.

• Fabrics: A certain tailorable weight and fall. Shape depends on how straight it falls from the shoulders. It must not collapse anywhere. Velvet, tweed, gabardine, and cotton duck work well. Watch out for a bad manufacturing trick of making the *lining* stiff to compensate for a limp outer fabric.

The Shirt Jacket

The "Safari Jacket" Shape is extremely popular in softer fabrics. Often unlined (less bulk), it is meant to be worn belted or unbelted. Think flannel, soft tweed, cotton, jersey . . . even silky fabrics! A handy warm weather version could be a shirt jacket in beige or navy shantung or silk-and-linen blend. Follow the jacket length rules for skirts and trousers.

• Classic length: ½″ *below* derriere; a slightly longer length than the square jacket as this shape becomes shorter when belted. *Therefore if you plan to wear it belted* test the length belted. If you plan to wear it loose, you will probably want to shorten the jacket—especially if you need leg length.

Cardigan

• A square straight-from-shoulder shape—usually collarless and buttonless. A very handy city jacket, as this shape moves easily over skirts and dresses! Fit is key:

• The curve of the collar must be in a smooth line, low enough in front so it grazes collar bone. If it moves up in front or sits too high on sides of neck or at back of neck, it is wrong!

• Stand straight. The jacket front should close edge to edge and fall die-straight (and *closed*) from neck to hem with no gaps or ripples anywhere!

• This length works best a bit shorter than the blazer length. Below hipbone to top of leg is the measure. A cardigan is not the ideal trouser jacket if you have a hip-derriere problem. However, it is a perfect trouser shape if it is ¾ (mid-thigh) or ⅞ (a hand-above-knee) long. It then becomes a fine coat length to wear over skirts and dresses.

• Fabrics: As with the square-shaped, collared jacket, the cardigan is best in fabrics with a "hand" as it must fall straight and not collapse anywhere: flat tweeds, shantung silk, linen, cotton canvas, satin for evening, etc. It is a "treasure" in velvet as it can work for day with flannel, tweed, and jersey and double as the indispensable evening jacket over anything!

• In the longer ¾ or ⅞ length one often finds this shape quilted.

SKIRTS

The Classics

REMEMBER: No matter what the skirt shape, waistbands should never bind! Aside from squeezing (and feeling terrible), a tight waist instantly knocks off the correct fit of skirt.

The straight (as opposed to A-line) wrap skirt is an investment!

• This shape looks good on most bodies as it is a slimming proportion.

• One can move in it easily.

• As opposed to A-line wrap, this shape is an investment—A most adaptable shape day to evening . . . a narrow wrap skirt in black cotton for summer, one in black wool or gabardine for winter. Make infinite day and evening looks. It's narrow, so you can wear tops over or tuck them in, depending on the look you want!

• Ideal length: just covering the point where the back of the calf curves into knee!

• When you buy a narrow wrap skirt make sure that it falls straight from waist to hem—if it angles in or out, it is out-of-kilter.

• Make sure wrap edge falls straight from waist to hem for the same reason.

The Eight Classic Skirt

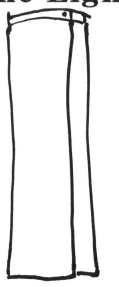

Straight Wrap

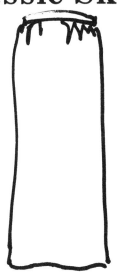

Eased Dirndl

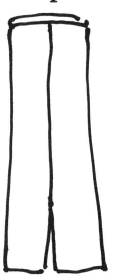

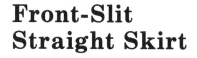

Front-Slit Straight Skirt

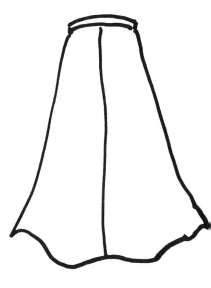

Bias Skirt

Shapes

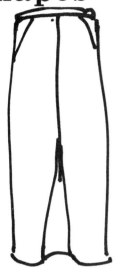

Front-Pleated

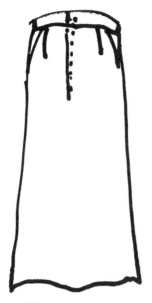

Trouser-Pleated

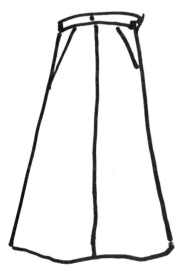

A-Line Skirt

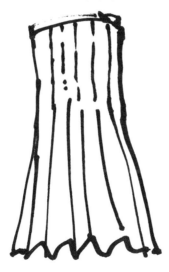

Hip-Stitched Pleated Skirt

• Make sure there is enough "wrap" so that when you walk or sit down you aren't "unwrapped"!

This shape works in most fabrics, although heavy wool or any bulky fabric will add pounds because of front double layer.

Eased dirndl

• A very flattering shape for most bodies although it can emphasize width of hips. The points to look for:

• Well-balanced gathers—not too full in any one spot—*especially not full at sides*! The best ones concentrate fullness a little more at center front and back and slightly *less* on sides to offset any emphasis on width of hips. The ones with ease only in front (with smooth sides and back) are ideal if you have big hip problems. Make sure sides and back fall straight and do not cling.

• The best fabrics for an eased dirndl: jersey or any *soft* fabrics (soft wool, cotton, silk, etc.) Stiff fabrics are usually too bulky—they can't take the subtle shirring at waist.

• Look for narrow waistbands: this is an instant waist and hip minimizer. If you can find this shape on a narrow *elastic* waistband (make sure fabrics are ultra-soft in this case!), it is even better, as this way you are never squeezed at waist.

• Since this shape is fuller, you can wear it a bit shorter than a plumb-straight skirt, especially for day, but *always covering the curve of calf into knee at the back of the leg*! Try it a bit longer for evening in silk or georgette. When the fabric is very floaty, it feels and looks so pretty flowing around the legs when you walk!

• Remember, this is a shape to tuck tops *into*. You can only wear tops over if they are loose enough to fall smoothly and not show skirt gathers!

Front-pleated skirt

(Sometimes made with a back pleat as well—same rules apply!)

• Slimming shape. For correct fit, it must fall *straight* at sides from waist to hem and when you are standing straight, with legs together, the pleats must close evenly all the way down.

• The fabric here is important. Heavy wools only work if they are balanced perfectly—they must fall plumb-straight. Watch out for very thin fabrics in this shape; unless they are artfully stitched, they risk looking "homemade." Never buy one in jersey—usually too limp to hold pleats.

• This shape works best in medium weight fabrics such as cotton, gabardine, wool, crepe, crêpe de chine. You can wear tops in or over, as the hip area is smooth.

Trouser-pleated skirt

Now as classic a shape as pleated trousers! There are even versions with a trouser-like front zipper.
• Wear it as one would a trouser—a great day easy-skirt-look! (Not a useful evening shape, although one in black wool could pass.)

• Here again—the key to proper fit is in side seams: They must fall straight from waist to hem.

• Waist should be as loose as possible as those little trouser pleats will instantly make a stomach-bulge. But, *if waist is loose and does not bind* and skirt falls straight and smooth to hem, this shape can be a stomach camouflager!

• Trouser-weight fabrics are best in this shape—ones with a "hand" (that is, fabrics with a tailorable weight) that aren't too limp (jersey) or too thin (silk). The best fabrics with a "hand"—flannel, gabardine, tweed, cotton duck, or soft cotton canvas. It is best to tuck tops into this skirt-shape. You might wear them out only if they are short enough to stop before pleats start, as in a short (2″ below waist) sweater or a blouse that is belted and bloused to stop at top of pleats.

• The length is important! The skirt must be long enough to cover the point where back of calf curves in to knee.

• If this shape is too short with all the "waist emphasis," one risks looking top-heavy. If it is too long, it is a definitely dowdy and draggy proportion.

Front-Slit Skirt

• This is a slimming shape, as it is narrow, but only if it *is* even and straight from waist to hem . . . it must never cling!

• The slit is a flattering leg-lengthener, as when you move, a bit of leg flashes through. However, make sure the slit is no deeper than 2″ above knee or you have an Apache-dancer costume!

• **LENGTH:** It must cover the part of back of calf that curves in towards knee. . . . If this shape is too short it will look vulgar *and* shorten your proportion, especially leg length!

• In thinner fabrics (jersey, crepe, etc.) it is a useful late-day shape. Great in tweed, flannel, even cotton duck for day as it is a smooth, slim, perfect shape *over* which to wear blouses, tunics or sweaters.

Trick: Collect this shape if you've a weight problem or a hip-stomach one. Then collect matching tops to slide over with ease. The best tops: tunic length, covering the behind! The effect: *instantly* slimming! Be sure to tone stocking and shoe to match skirt for maximum slimming and proportion lengthening.

Bias Skirt

• This shape works best in soft fabrics that move: thin wool, or silk jersey, silk, rayon, thin cotton, crepe. It can be heavy and stiff in any fabric with weight!

• A pretty summer-day and any season late-day shape (although a medium-full bias skirt in navy or beige wool jersey is a perfect *day* skirt anytime). It depends entirely on the amount of bias fullness *and* on the fabric! Guide: less bias in a day fabric, more for evening or easy summer country day (a gauzy one!). Look carefully at seams to make sure there is no puckering, as bias fabric is often difficult to sew.

• Remember: the nature of bias means cling—and it *does*, across stomach and hips. If you want to camouflage these

areas this may NOT be the shape for you! (If however, the skirt is *not too full* and you can *slide a top over* it to the area where the fullness begins around the thigh, you might make it work—but it's tricky!)

• This shape in thin floaty fabrics (georgette, thin silk, cotton gauze, thin stocking weight jersey, etc.) is lovely to wear a bit longer for evening (even midcalf if you've the leg length, as the bias makes floaty fabric even floatier!

A-Line —The Neat Basic Shape

• Best for day in jean fabric, cotton canvas, etc.—or rough country tweed. Often this shape exists as a wrap. Again, it is best in daytime jeans-like or tweedy fabrics.

• It's not particularly interesting as an evening or city dressing shape. Usually designers choose one of the other seven around which to work their important statements. This shape is handy and nice if used in a very country way: with a cotton T-shirt, a Shetland sweater, and shirt, espadrilles or loafers, and woolly stockings.

Hip-Stitched Pleated Skirt

—often done with pleats and stitching in front panel only—

back of skirt falling smooth and straight.

• If you have hip-stomach problems it is not for you.

• Great elongating shape, however, as there is so much vertical emphasis.

• Look for a perfect straight line waist-to-hem, and most important—when you stand straight, legs together—that *all* pleats close plumb-straight and smooth. You can wear tops in or out (as stitched-down hip area is flat).

• This shape is prettiest in softer fabrics (the more pleats, the softer the fabric should be the rule!)—thin wool, silk/wool blends, crepe, gabardine, silk. It is not good for limp fabrics such as jersey.

• A good day-into-evening shape: a navy or black thin wool crepe version can work day and evening all year round!

• The nice part of wearing this shape is the movement of the pleats when you walk. As the fabrics become thinner, the length can become a little longer as the "float" of fabric around legs is flattering. The perfect length for day and evening: never shorter than where back of calf curves into back of knee!

PANTS

The Four Classic Shapes

Flat Pant

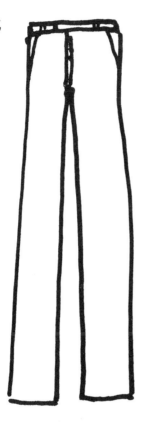

Pleated Trousers

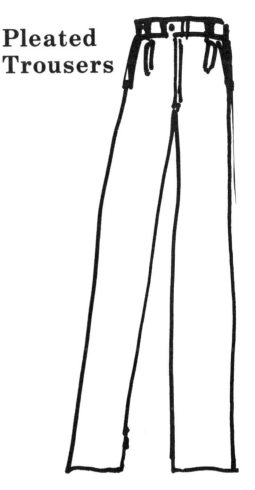

GENERAL RULE: *Look for straight legs*—the *illusion* of same width top-to-bottom. Classic. Bottom width 17″–19″. (The rule followed for well-tailored men's pants.)

• **Note 1:** The illusion of a die-straight leg is best attained when bottom width of leg is slightly *narrower* than knee width. The knee measures about 19″–20″ and from there down lessens gradually to 17″–19″.

• **Note 2:** Trouser leg widths move in and out quickly from season to season. Keeping within this conservative range insures longest life!

• General rule for length: Pants bottom should hit top of shoe and then "break" slightly so that *when you walk* it still hits top of shoe. When measuring length be sure to walk around! Length should be *even* all around—should never dip and angle down at back. No matter what anyone says, pants should *not* be longer in back. Be sure to determine a *basic shoe height* for your pants. The way to keep pants

Pull-On Elastic Waist Pajama

Jeans

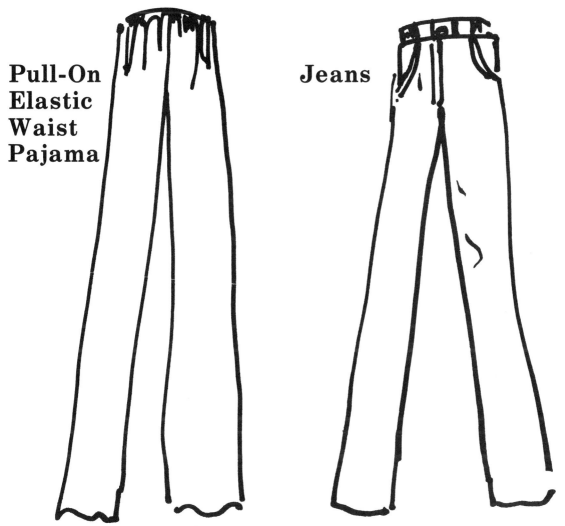

working well for you is to decide *where* you will wear them mostly—to work, in the country, to dinner as well as to work? Then ask yourself what shoe height you will be wearing mostly—flat moccasins (country), medium heel (day), higher heels (night)? This all takes careful planning *and* shoe shopping! See shoe section for tips.

• General Length Pants Rule: *Measure trouser length to "day shoe"* and then go ⅛" longer or shorter depending on the "secondary shoe" height.

• Pants over bare sandals can be a *bit* shorter than with a more serious day shoe. Remember, we are speaking of fractions of an inch!

• For more leg length: Leave off all cuffs.

• Pants waistbands should never be too wide. One inch is ideal. They should sit comfortably *at waist* and never bind.

• Watch out for pants with waistbands that sit *below* natural waist; they are instantly leg shorteners. The *higher* the illusion of waist, the *longer* the illusion of leg!

• If you *are short-waisted* you may, however, *want* to lower the waistline of pants to graze *just below* your natural waistline to give the **illusion** of a longer torso. Don't sacrifice leg length if you do. A careful study in a full-length three-way mirror is vital.

• Take a long look at your back view in a three-way mirror (so that you get the best direct angle.) Remember, pockets accent hips and derriere! Back yokes and stitching (most often found on jeans) accent hips and derriere. No matter what your shape, make absolutely sure trousers or pants are *never tight* across your behind. Better a little on the loose side—looks trimmer, neater *and* trousers will fall straighter and more attractively!

• In general: Check total silhouette. Pants should hang straight, waist to foot, and never pucker along seams or ride up in crotch. Smooth and straight is the look! Fly-front closures should lie flat, never pull or pucker. Zippers should be totally invisible.

Flat Pant

• The best cut is like a man's —natural waist, fly front, beltloops, side pockets.

• Stay away from fancy details such as top-stitching, back yokes, fancy back pockets. As it is so pure and simple, this is a difficult shape to tailor well. Therefore, tricky details are often used to mask faults!

• This is a great shape for lengthening the silhouette (one long line)! You can easily wear tops tucked in or pulled over, as there is no extra fabric (such as pleats) to break the smooth line. If you have hips, stomach, or derriere to hide, this is the shape for you. Wear tunic tops over, making sure they hit mid-thigh—good camouflage!

FABRICS: anything from tweed to shantung silk. Overly thin silk is usually too soft to take the tailoring of a fly-front zipper.

• A great shape day and *evening* . . . A pair of flat-front pants in brown velvet or black gabardine can work wonders in a wardrobe as you can tuck tops in or wear them over. This is such a simple pants shape you can add and subtract accessories for dozens of looks and uses.

Pleated Trousers

• Another great classic shape, These can be a hip emphasizer because of pleats but a boon to a bit-of-stomach if the trousers fit a little on the loose side and

the pleats lie *flat* and face inward, to hide a little bulge!

• The best are cut like a man's, with a natural waist, fly front, beltloops, and side pockets. Make sure the pockets angle a tiny bit if you want to *minimize hip emphasis*. When pockets run directly along side seam up and down, they give the illusion of more hip, adding another layer of fabric where less fabric matters!

KEY: Pleats should never pull open nor look skimpy (as in: "Are they really meant to be there?"). Pleats should fall neatly, and the trouser leg should fall straight without any interference from pleats.

• This is a super shape to tuck shirts and pullovers into. You can wear tops out, *provided they stop above pleats* (i.e., short-waisted sweaters). Loose silk or jersey tops or tunics will work worn over provided they are *loose enough to fall smoothly over the pleats*. Watch out for anything that clings—it will accent stomach and show pleats!

• Pleated trousers are a great day shape. They will work for "easy" evenings (small restaurants, movies, drinks at someone's home, etc.), if you don't try to make them too formal!

FABRICS: Tweeds, flannel,

cotton, gabardine, corduroy, velvet, etc. Stay away from very thin silk (unless shantung), clingy or droopy fabrics unless they are cut *expertly*. There are too many details in this trouser for thin fabrics!

Elastic Pull-On Pants (The pajama)

• The sophisticated version of drawstring pants (in inexpensive cotton gauze and rayony fabrics found in Indian shops—so fabulous for summer!) They are best in evening or thin day fabrics.

• The key to fit: not too much shirring of fabric around elastic so that when worn the elastic flattens and there isn't an excess of fabric around waist and hips. *Neat fit is key!*

• Make sure the side and inseams hang straight and do not pucker as these pants are usually made in thin fabrics which take more care when being sewn!

• Make sure they sit properly at the crotch—neither riding up nor hanging too low—as perfect shape is key for this relatively unconstructed pant.

• Great for most bodies. They are slimming, especially with tunics or overtops. Be careful if you plan to tuck tops in or wear short tops out that *don't*

come below derriere since this shape is unconstructed and therefore very revealing!

FABRICS: Jersey, knit of any type, silk, thin cotton, thin silky velvet, wool, crepe, satin, any fabric that takes shirring easily! In wool and gabardine, be extra sure of the fit as these are basically fabrics for constructed pants.

• Collect elastic waist pants in silky fabrics. They are endlessly useful as instant-evening looks.

• Find: A navy, silky shantung "pajama" is great for warm climates (city, resort, etc.). Add a navy T-shirt and heeled sandals—a hot-city-day uniform! Wear espadrilles and you are set for a resort area or the country!

Jeans

KEY: Buy classic and wear classic! No matter what the ads say, never overly tight in behind! If you're sixteen and *perfect* . . . maybe, and just maybe! But the girdle, poured-in effect looks awful on most bodies, any age. Straight, slim, and neat are key.

• Well-washed is essential especially if blue denim. Nothing looks less easy than new jeans—and the look of jeans should be unobtrusive and

easy above all!

• Stay away from unclassic ones with too much stitching, too many labels, any tricky details! The best jeans are the classics like Levi's or Lee's. Save cut-off edges and patches for your twelve-year old child!

FABRICS: Best in traditional jeans fabric—denim, corduroy, cotton twill, drill, cotton canvas, thin cotton poplin for warm-weather wear. Velveteen works if made well but works best on young bodies.

• Stay away from trick fabrications; there never was a need for gray flannel jeans, and there never was a pair that looked right!

• Jeans should not be pretentious. They are useful and fabulous-looking for easy day and *very* easy country-evening. Nothing beats well-washed and trim jeans, a great Shetland sweater, tweed jacket and well-polished low heeled boots for the best country look American-style!

• However, if you don't look long and lean in jeans, *don't wear them*! (Or if you do, wear them only for painting your bedroom!) Opt instead for proper trousers of blue denim, corduroy or cotton drill, or wear a skirt of jeans fabric instead.

DRESSES

This book is about building a wardrobe around pieces—that is, skirts, trousers, jackets, sweaters, blouses, and accessories—with a relationship to each other, a consistent style and mobility so that a few pieces become numberless, interchangeable looks—and looks which *work for you*! If you follow this guide and build a wardrobe around pieces, your day and evening *basic needs* are taken care of. However, there is a moment when dressing requires a real *dress*! It may be your mood. It may be the occasion. It may be the availability of wonderful dresses after seasons of never finding any great ones. Remember: as these dresses are *additions to your wardrobe*, they should make you *feel* and *look* wonderful as well as perform successfully! Otherwise pass until you find ones that do. Choose them carefully. They should move into your Basic Wardrobe easily and work with the day and night pieces you already own!

General Rule: Think proportion. Think tone. Think beautiful fabrics.

The 4 Basic Dress Shapes

Shirtdress

Wrap dress

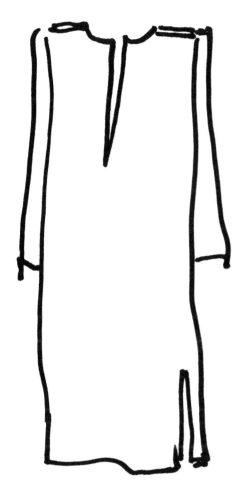

Chemise or
Tunic Dress

(Classic caftan shape—wear
loose or blouse and belt)

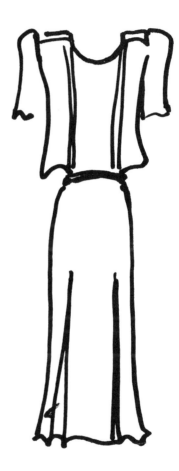

Dresses with
a Defined
Waist

DRESSES

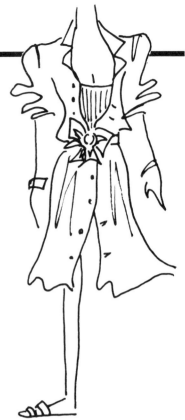

Shirtdress

• **Shape:** The most useful is cut straight from shoulder to hem. (See Basic Wardrobe, Blouses. Follow the same guidelines.) Collars and cuffs should have no stiffening in them; soft is key. Details: as unadorned as possible—minimum stitching, few pockets, buttons, always toned to dress color, etc. Small, simple four-hole buttons are best.

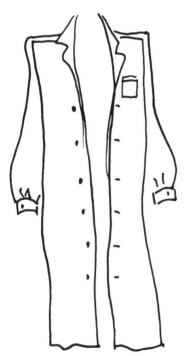

•**FABRICS:** The best fabrics, soft.—silk, jersey, cotton knit, thin cotton, linen, thin thin soft wool or blends of wool and silk, etc. . . . Fabrics that *move* attractively and can play a *seasonless role.*

• *Changing accessories changes the look.* For example: Belt a Bordeaux silk shirtdress in pigskin for day. To change the look for night, belt in black satin and wear unbuttoned to the waist with a little black silk camisole underneath. Add pretty sparkle jewelry. Slide a tweed jacket over a silky shirtdress for an autumn day, a velvet jacket at night for dinner, a linen or cotton jacket in summer . . . Wear the same silk shirtdress unbuttoned and belted over a sweater for work in winter . . . belt it with a cotton scarf and wear over a bare T-shirt in summer with flat canvas sandals!

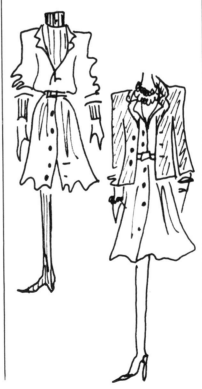

• A shirtdress is a universal shape. Most body proportions can wear it as long as there is a *minimum amount of fullness* above and below waist when belted. This fullness is controlled by the width of dress shoulder to hem. It could be a question of slimming only ½″ to 1″ at each side to make it work for you!

•If you are big-hipped or very overweight, you might choose a straight tunic-shaped dress instead of risking that squeezed-in-the-middle look or wear a shirtdress loose, silky, and straight! Make sure the length is flattering to your leg and proportion. This is a great shape if you are tall and slim, the blousier the better!

TRICK: If it is well cut—straight, soft, and beautiful—it can double as a coat! In summer, slide a taupe silk shirtdress over a bare black T-shirt and black cotton pants and wear it as a silky "cover". Add sandals—peanut leather for day, gold for night—fabulous look!

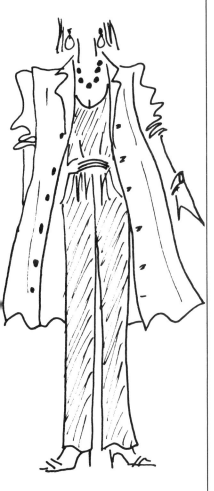

Wrap Dress

•The most useful come with separate belts rather than the attached ones that pull dress closed, go through a slit in side, and then wrap. Although it's more difficult to find the right amount to wrap over, to blouse a *tiny* bit and to arrange the fall of the fabric, this unbelted version insures a slimmer-proportioned dress after being closed and belted. The type that has an attached belt usually has a fuller-gored skirt. Added bonus: With the do-it-yourself-closing, *you can change* belts! This means day/evening/winter/summer. A wardrobe treasure.

KEY: Thin, soft fabrics (our usual list) toned to your basic wardrobe.

•Major concern: The amount of wrapover! Make sure that when you walk and sit you have no surprises—the wrapover and wrapunder should be ample enough to allow you to move freely without suddenly finding yourself nearly undressed! This shape comes with short sleeves, long sleeves—even sleeveless (especially pretty in thin linen)—with narrow notched collars, shawl collars, or no collars at all, just a good, flat V-wrapped line. *All* these work well in solid colors or pretty small prints and geometrics.

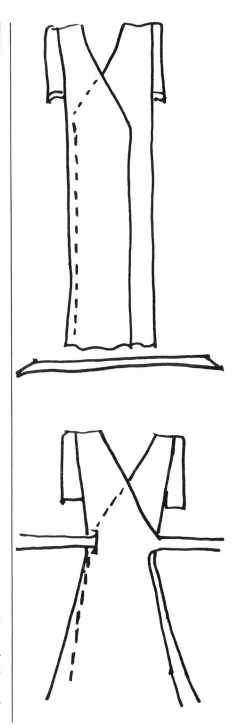

DRESSES

•Tip: Think about the jackets, cardigans, and silky coverings in your wardrobe and choose colors and patterns with those in mind! A thin linen wrap-dress in caramel is perfect to wear under a tan, navy, or white linen or cotton jacket with peanut leather accessories to go to work/city or add a dark rose canvas belt, rose-and-tan cream cotton scarf at neck, pale tan flat sandals, and you have a great resort look perfect for lunch, tennis matches, etc. Or add a hemp rope at the waist and espadrilles, and you have an easy Summer Country look. A big straw shoulder bag to make the turnout extra summery and attractive!

•**More ways to wear a Wrap Dress: Trick for summer:** Open the top more than usual and wear a bare T-shirt camisole under! A dark ground print silk (e.g., black with a tiny tan check) plus a jacket in brown tweed = Autumn Day. Add a jacket in black velvet and you have a perfect dinner look; a jacket in cocoa linen, summer! Slide a black silk strapless camisole underneath and wear it opened to the waist—great

Dinner Dressing! This dress is a treasure! A pretty, skin-color, pale tone of silk can be the dress that saves your life for any number of last-minute weddings/black-tie suppers/cocktail party situations. One of black silk satin or jacquarded silk can do for nearly any city dressy evening except for a big-time black-tie formal one!

•Wrapdresses work for most body proportions. If, however, you have a *big bosom* problem or *extra broad shoulders—pass*. The nature of the crisscross closing of top emphasizes bosom and the horizontal line of shoulders!

• It's a *great* shape for *short necks* and *small bosoms* because the open neck reveals skin—lengthening the neck. The crisscross line gives the illusion of more bosom.

• If you have *big hips and a wide waist: Do* look for the do-it-yourself wrap kind. Use a narrow-toned belt or matching fabric string tie to close the dress. Make sure there is never but the *tiniest* amount of blousing over the belt and that the dress wraps as smoothly and narrowly as possible! The off-center wrap then becomes a very slimming line. Make sure, however, that the back of the dress falls straight and smoothly with just a little ease at midcenter back!

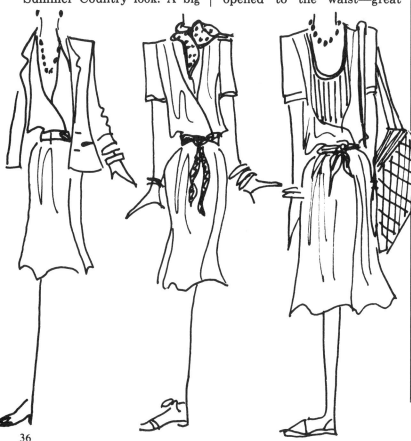

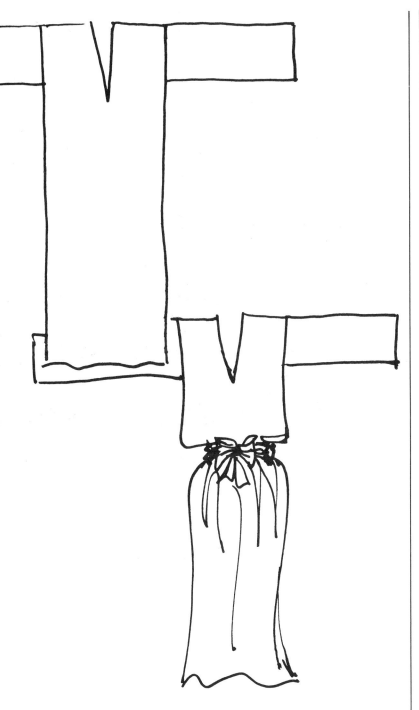

(The classic caftan shape)

• *A straight line is key.* This shape is meant to be worn loose from shoulder to hem (not a tenty A-line shape! See "3B" for A-line version). It can also be worn waist-tied or belted with a bit of easy blousing over belt and a little gathering below belt.

• Again, thin, soft fabrics are best—silk, thin wool, cotton, or blends of wool and silk, jersey, crepe de chine, woven silk such as shantung, twill, etc., knitted wool, cashmere, cotton knit, even soft cotton and gauze.

Shape details: You will find endless detail variations— sleeveless, strapless, bare camisole tops; long sleeves such as shirtsleeves; loose straight kimonos or caftanlike sleeves; narrow straight sleeves; short, set-in or raglan sleeves, etc. Necklines can be bare or V, round (high or low), with or without collars, slitneck, or button-front shirtcollars. This shape is found plain with gathers, pleats, or tucks at shoulder seam—in other words, there are endless variations. Know your figure and proportion needs and you can find the *perfect* one for you!

DRESSES

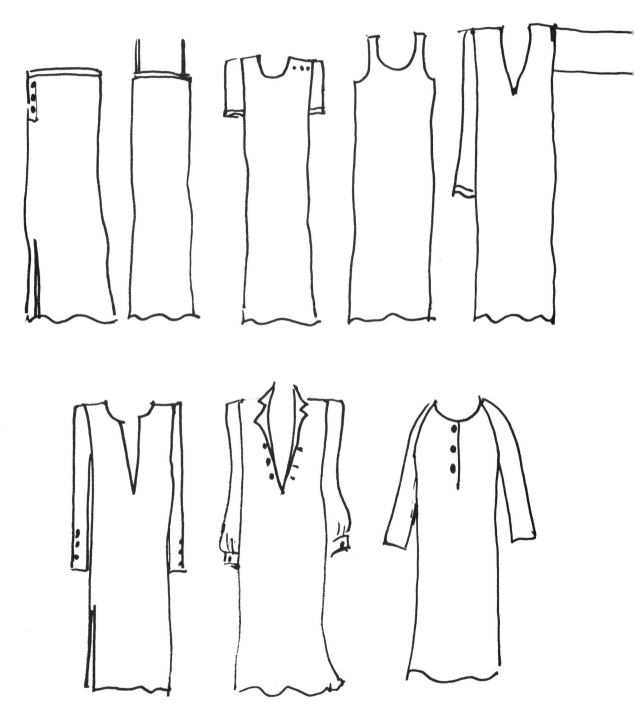

To search for:

• **_The Perfect Evening Treasure:_** A "covered" version of chemise-tunic shape in a soft, beautiful silk or jacquard silk. For example, long pretty sleeves, a slit neckline to show a bit of skin or a round neckline with a tiny covered button to close when you want to be proper and to open for allure! The point: A _subtly chic_ version that becomes the _universal dress_ to wear when you're not sure what is safe and you want to look your best! Wear it at night anywhere in the world—summer or winter. _It is always right._ Do your best hair, prettiest makeup, perfect jewelry and voilá... it's safe, chic, and _very attractive_!

• Note: Because you can wear this shape _unbelted_, it is _the_ perfect dress shape for overweight or big derriere/hip problems! In silky fabrics that _do not cling_ and fall _softly_ over the body _barely_ skimming the _widest_ parts, there is no better shape. It masks perfectly and is flattering! A wine crepe de chine tunic dress with bare camisole or carved top, a peanut belt and sandals, plus navy linen cardigan = Summer City/Day. Waist-tied with a black velvet ribbon plus black velvet jacket = Autumn City/Evening. It is a perfect business, dinner, theatre, or cocktail-party look. Worn bloused over narrow black silk pajamas, a fabulous dinner-party look!

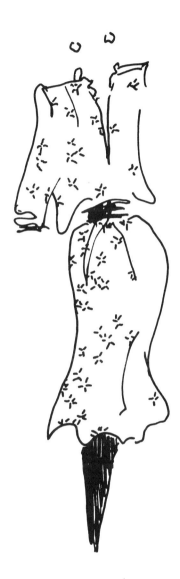

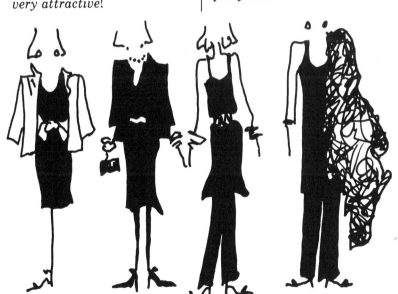

• Work   • City Dinner   • Dinner, private home or drinks at club

• **_Overweight trick:_** Wear it loose if you have hips! Trick: Add big black silk or thin cashmere shawl to distract even more! Remember: match stocking and shoe color to dress.

DRESSES

To collect:

• **Perfect Day Treasure:**
The same dress in a soft jersey or thin wool (or silk for warm places), dark-toned, long-sleeved (to roll), with an easy pretty neckline (open collar, round, V, slit, etc.). They will take you to conference lunches, meetings, appointments—anywhere you have to look poised, pulled together, businesslike, conservative, and *attractively all of these!*

A-Line Tent Dress

• There is a version of a loose-shaped dress which begins small at the top and moves *gently* out into an A- or tent-triangle shape. This is *perfect camouflage* for weight problems provided you are small on top: narrow rather than broad shoulders, not-too-big bosomed, dnd, if dress sleeves are set in, not too heavy in arms! It is the universal shape for maternity dresses (as well as the straight chemise-tunic).

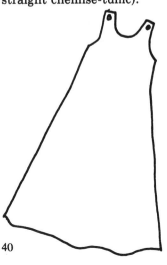

• The A-line is a very flattering shape for small, short-proportioned bodies, especially in delicate silky fabrics: thin silk, jersey, knit, cotton gauze, etc., which float gracefully *near* the body. *Never stiff fabrics* or one risks looking as if literally in a tent or between sandwich boards!

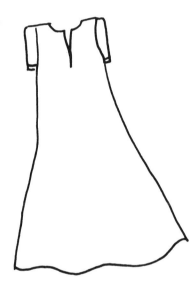

• The nature of the A-line is good for small, delicate figures: the top is close to the body and the line moves out so gently one never looks swamped in too much fabric! For variation, you can waist-tie this shape, but only if it is not *too* triangular or you will wind up with too much skirt after you belt! Try belting only if the dress is in a silky fabric and then only with a narrow string-of-a-belt.

• As soon as there is a cut at the waist—a seam, the place where the top and the skirt attach—anything can happen. The waist definition can be as simple as an elastic and give the same effect as your chemise-tunic shape when you belt it. Variations: Big top, slim skirt . . . Narrow top, full skirt . . . Big top, big skirt.

To wear this shape:

• Know your proportion/figure problems and figure assets—what works and what does not work. Know also that these dresses are usually less classic, more fashion-oriented, and fashion-determined; therefore less movable, less seasonless, and less useful. That is not to say, however, less desirable!

Category I—Practical

• In the classic "working-for-you" sense these defined waistdresses could be another variation on a soft, easy dress which works into your Basic Wardrobe and lifestyle perfectly—attractive, handy, movable and usable with what you already own and *delightful to wear*! These are shapes in which attractive dinner dresses as well as day/work/meeting looks can be found. *They become collectibles.*

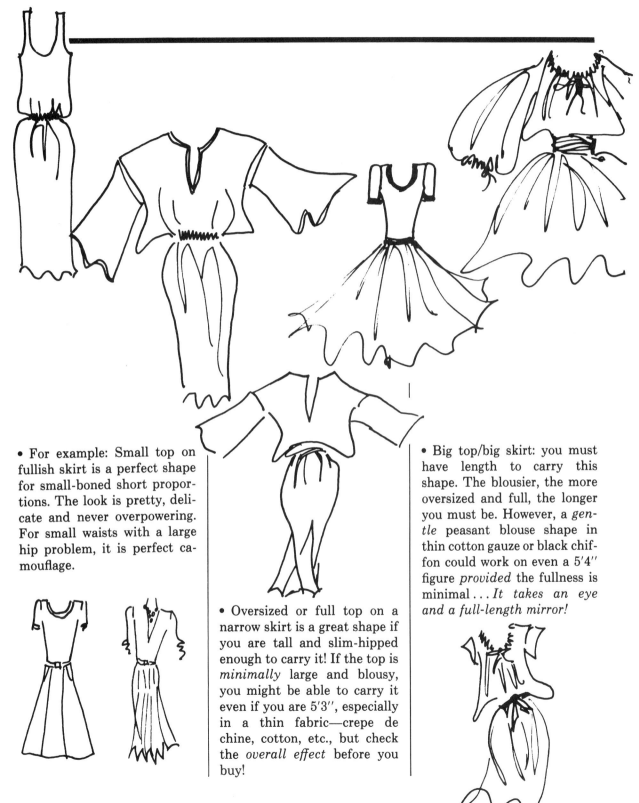

• For example: Small top on fullish skirt is a perfect shape for small-boned short proportions. The look is pretty, delicate and never overpowering. For small waists with a large hip problem, it is perfect camouflage.

• Oversized or full top on a narrow skirt is a great shape if you are tall and slim-hipped enough to carry it! If the top is *minimally* large and blousy, you might be able to carry it even if you are 5′3″, especially in a thin fabric—crepe de chine, cotton, etc., but check the *overall effect* before you buy!

• Big top/big skirt: you must have length to carry this shape. The blousier, the more oversized and full, the longer you must be. However, a *gentle* peasant blouse shape in thin cotton gauze or black chiffon could work on even a 5′4″ figure *provided* the fullness is minimal ... *It takes an eye and a full-length mirror!*

DRESSES

• Small top/big top and very full skirts/narrow skirts . . . *evening dressing!* Follow the same rules!

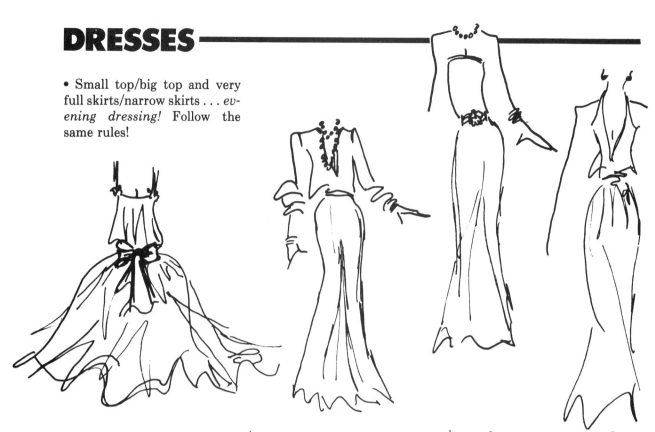

Category II—Special Occasion Dresses

• These are dresses you buy because you need something perfect to wear to one or more major social event: the opening of the opera, your best friend's wedding, a black-tie dinner at the home of your husband's boss, a testimonial dinner where you will receive an award, etc.

• Or there are dresses which are *whims!* You buy because you see the dress you've always longed to have (a white silk organza strapless dance dress, a washed-peach cotton gauze calf-long peasant dress, a floor-length sarong-dress of black hammered satin, a wisp of a pale mauve chiffon halter dress with a skirt that moves like a dancer in a summer breeze . . . poetry! The events will come later.

• *Danger:* These are the dresses, or purchases in general, to watch out for. They are delights, alluring, beautiful, etc. *They could be extravagances also!* Don't buy them when you are rushed or frazzled. If you need a dress for next week's opera opening, relax, pull yourself together, organize, *reread the section on How To Shop!* Then start looking. If, on the other hand, you pass a window with the peach gauze peasant dress, walk past it two or three blocks! Then, if you turn around and walk back, justify that whim by knowing:

1. That it *is* your style—not a 40-year-old's fantasy of what it was like to be 16!
2. That it works perfectly with your proportion/figure problems (honestly).
3. That it looks wonderful— really spectacular—and makes you feel beautiful!
4. That "cross-your-heart-" you will have somewhere to wear it . . . you are going to Majorca in two months' time or your best friend *really* is getting married in July . . .
5. That it is affordable. Otherwise, walk on!

COATS

- A *coat is a major investment*. Buy the best you can afford! This means best fabric, better workmanship, better fit, longest life.

- Remember: *No one coat will meet all your needs* (from jeans to major-evening dressing). There is no point in looking for it or expecting your choice to do 100 percent duty! Therefore *analyze your priorities* and aim for the coat that will serve them in the best way possible.

- Analyze your closet. What is your basic color family? Black is a basic for some, but if you dress predominately in browns and beiges your neutral coat color might be vicuña or milk chocolate brown.

- What do you wear most? Trousers, skirts, or dresses? A fitted coat is great over skirts but you won't want to wear it for trouser-dressing.

- Analyze what your daily routine is. If you work in an office you will want to look businesslike. If you spend your time keeping house and children, a tweed coat will serve almost every day. If you travel, drive a lot, or commute, you will want a practical coat ... perhaps a ⅞ shape for ease in and out of cars. Do you need to look dressed for day? Do you attend a lot of lunches, meet-

ings? Do you have an extensive nightlife? In the country? City? Warm or changeable temperature?

- Analyze your body.

- Do you have hip problems? You will *not* want a narrow bathrobe wrapcoat or *anything* that ties at the waist! Are you short? Simple shapes, minimum detail are best (no epauletted trenchcoats or raglan-sleeved shapes that risk looking top-heavy. Look for narrow rather than wide shapes. Do you have a short neck or big bosom? Look for neat open collars or none . . . never a coat that needs to close high at the neck.

- *General rule: Simple is best*. Stay away from anything over-detailed: big fancy buttons, too much stitching, too many yokes, panels, pocket flaps with decoration, too many pockets, too many buttons (on sleeves, epaulets, pockets, down the front). Often manufacturers try to give you your money's worth by adding on all but the proverbial kitchen sink!

- *Length*: Your coat should cover your skirt length by ½″. This way the skirt hem won't peek out when you walk and the coat moves. However, for economy's sake don't fall into the trap of keeping it longer

than you need so that you can wear it for more seasons. This is false economy. Your coat will always look wrong, feel wrong and look dowdy!

- *Sleeve length*: For the fit of collar, shoulders, etc., see Jacket Section. Remember: The secret of the fit of a coat is *balance*. It should hang evenly, comfortably and straight from your shoulders and *never* feel heavy across the shoulders. If it does, it can be painful after hours of wear and is clearly a sign of something wrong in the fit!

- The front opening should hang evenly closed when you stand straight, legs together. The same goes for any back vent or pleat detail. Pockets should lie flat, never pull or gape open. You should be able to raise your arms easily without feeling resistance.

- *Remember*: Think carefully about what you will wear *under* your coat. If you wear a lot of jackets try your coat on with a jacket underneath. Can you move easily in it without looking overstuffed? If you wear your coat mainly over sweaters, blouses, or thin dresses you do not want to look "drowned" in it; you want it to fit more closely, like a jacket.

- Check that linings aren't too stiff or fight the coat fabric

The Five Classic Coat Shapes

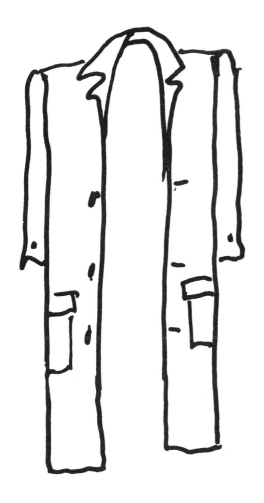

Straight Overcoat

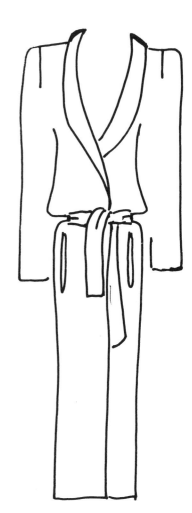

**Narrow-Wrap
Bathrobe
Coat**

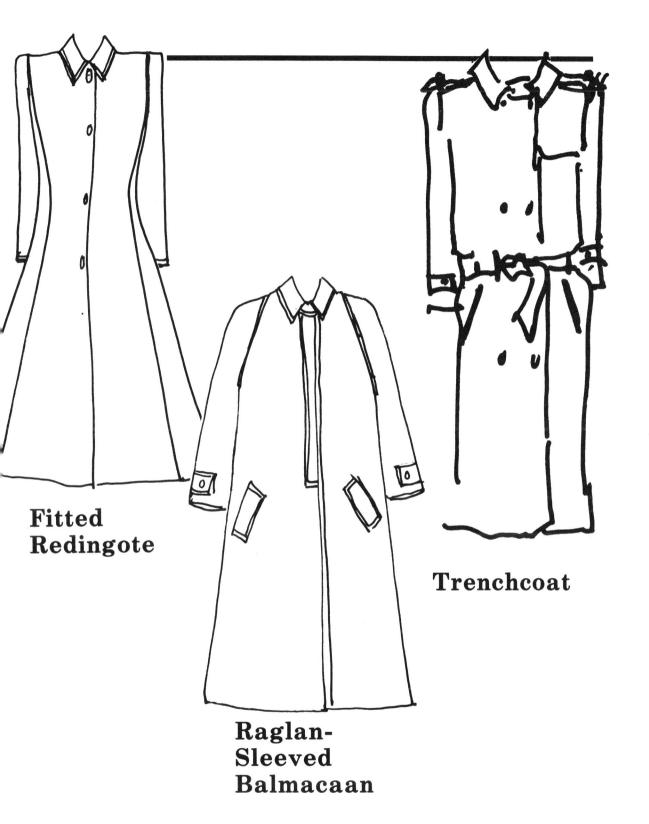

**Fitted
Redingote**

**Raglan-
Sleeved
Balmacaan**

Trenchcoat

(pull in the wrong direction). The ideal linings in certain coats (raincoats, thin gabardine ones, etc.) are button-out linings. Look for them as they make a coat seasonless—to wear in winter, spring, or fall.

Straight Classic Overcoat

• This is a versatile coat shape which can be worn easily over trousers as well as dresses and skirts. A straight, simple shape, it is relatively easy to wear for most proportions. Look for single-breasted ones for the same reason as you would a jacket: When you wear it open, there is less fabric. It hangs better!

• Make sure coat lapels are not extreme—that is, too wide or too narrow. 2½″ is a good median.

• The hang of this shape is key. It is a straight shape; it must fall straight and even shoulder-to-hem and not pitch forward or backward. Look carefully at your side view to make sure it falls vertically and evenly straight.

KEY: Search for models that are narrow rather than oversized or this shape could look as if you borrowed it from your father!

FABRICS: cashmere, soft wool (in camel, navy, black, etc., like a man's overcoat), tweed . . . Think classic tones and simple classic fabrics. This is a day shape although a black cashmere-and-wool overcoat could pass for easy-evening— for going to a local restaurant, movie, etc., when you are wearing trousers and a sweater, pretty jewelry. Never try to make it do too much evening duty or you risk looking like the girl with her camel hair coat over her prom dress! A great coat for city work and country.

Wrap Bathrobe Coat

• This shape requires wrapping and belting so it accents hips and derriere and weight problems! But if you can carry it, this is one of the most versatile shapes of all six basic coats. It works over skirts and dresses as well as pants. It can move easily from day to evening, depending on the fabric. A soft wool in a dark solid color is the Almost-Perfect Coat. Although it is more of a city shape, one of soft tweed or tan gabardine would work in the country without looking too dressy!

KEY: Make sure the fabric is supple as everything depends on how softly (and nonbulkily) this coat wraps and ties! Fabrics: soft wool, cashmere, jersey, gabardine, corduroy, twill, thin weights of tweed. Look for unlined versions—they are the wrappiest and least bulky—or ones with soft silky linings.

• Collar Variations: shawl-collared or knotched-collared. Either is fine, depending on your preference, provided that neither is too extreme in width!

Shoulder variations: set-in sleeves or raglan sleeves. If you want a "lift" to your proportion, opt for the set-in sleeve. If you are particularly broad-shouldered or tall and don't want to accentuate your height, opt for the raglan.

• A soft black or navy wool bathrobe coat can easily be your evening coat for short dresses or silky pajama dressing! A cream soft wool one is ideal for warmer places but obviously less handy for day. A vicuña-colored one is perfect if your color family for either day and evening is brown-toned.

NOTE: This shape works well as a ⅞ length (a hand above the knee). If you have the body—(no hip/derriere problems or extra weight)—this length will go easily over trousers, skirts and *long* slim dresses . . . again depending on fabric and color. It is a terrific fur shape. In fur you can wear it *unbelted*, which allows for camouflaging problem figures!

Fitted Redingote Coat

• The most feminine shape of all, it is great on short figures, especially if the curve of the waist hits just *above* your natural waist to make your legs look longer! The length must be perfect, for one tends to wear this shape as one would a dress; that is, *closed*. Ideally it should graze the leg perfectly or it risks looking draggy and dowdy.

• Watch out for Redingotes with too-full skirts. You do not want a skating-skirt look!

• As this shape is usually designed to button to the neck (rather than with a shawl or knotched collar), you might look "choked" if you have a short neck or big bosom.

• Look for the fewest and simplest details possible as this is one of the shapes that risks being "overdesigned"!

FABRICS: the best are those which take tailoring easily: thin tweeds, gabardine, soft wools, etc.

• This is definitely a *skirt or dress shape*. Unless worn expertly and perfectly balanced and toned over skinny pants for late day, it looks wrong with pants! It is a city shape, a feminine shape, a bit too dressy for country living.

• A redingote works well both day and evening depending on the fabric and color. A black or brown velvet one would be a super extra coat to wear over most short-dressing at night!

The Raglan Balmacaan

• A loose and slightly A-shaped coat. Although it is good for most bodies, if you are short you risk being swamped by the raglan sleeve, unless this shape is cut on the slim side. This is definitely *a sport-day shape*. If you dress in pants a lot for evening, a velvet one can be a handy *extra coat*. A Balmacaan works very well as a ¾ (mid-thigh) and ⅞ (hand-above-knee) coat shape. If you are short, these two lengths are great as you don't look "swamped." Again, think sport: tweed-lined poplin or thin leather, gabardine, Harris tweed, etc. A ⅞ or ¾ Balmacaan is the perfect country-suburban living coat—just right for a car life!

FABRICS: The Balmacaan is a traditional poplin raincoat shape. It is a treasure if you can find one with a button-out lining of wool or fake fur (alpaca). It then becomes a *seasonless* weather coat, ideal for winter, spring, fall, travel, etc.

• This shape is perfect to wear over jackets, heavy sweaters, etc. The raglan leaves room for underneath bulk.

• A handy city day and country shape, it works well over both skirts and trousers.

• It is clearly *not* a dress coat unless acting as a weather raincoat (or velvet).

• Best in classic fabrics such as tweed, camel's hair, gabardine, cotton poplin, leather . . . A great, easy fur-coat shape.

Trenchcoat

• Watch out for details, the traditional ones such as epaulettes, back yoke, shoulder patch must be classic and balanced. Fashiony ones such as too much stitching, extra bits of flaps and pieces of metal, etc. . . . pass on them! If you buy a trenchcoat buy a *real* one. Otherwise you are not buying a trenchcoat!

• If you have broad shoulders remove any epaulettes; your neighborhood tailor can do this.

• This classic raincoat shape works best in tan poplin or gabardine as a "weather" coat (especially handy with a button-out wool lining!).

• Trenchcoat versions are found in all fabrics, but the traditional poplin or gabardine "investment" will stay in your wardrobe forever, never look "fashiony" and therefore never dated!

BEAUTY ORGANIZATION

The Key: You! ... Your Body, Your Skin, Your Hair, Your Makeup. The Goal: The Best Total Picture Head to Toe!

THE BASIS: A Beauty/Health routine as efficient and as effective as possible.

Important: Beauty/Health Rituals Must Be Pleasing.

They are designed to make you look and feel better! They must be attractive and inviting to perform. *Organize. Begin with all the necessary tools.*
• Keep tools wonderfully *attractive*. Half the fun and effectiveness of beauty/health routines is the *pleasure!* Pretty tools, brushes, cases, an attractive leotard for exercise, pretty bottles of skin-care products and colognes and oils that look, feel, and smell nice! AND WORK!

Organize: Divide and Arrange!

• **Keep makeup** in pretty printed cotton bags or covered wicker or straw baskets.

• *Keep skin-treatment products* in other printed cotton bags or straw boxes. Cotton, Q-tips, tissues, etc. Antique silver covered powder boxes, pretty straw containers.

• **Have a *small, pretty tray* handy on which to lay out all your "tools" before beginning makeup.** It can be wicker or clear Lucite or silver . . . one of those "never-found-a-use-for" presents! **Tip:** *A tray is a* perfect way to move essentials around to good sources of making-up light. No one ever said makeup has to be done in the bathroom! For example: Check your living room window area for great daylight light. Do day makeup there—*it is the light in which you will be seen!* **Never do makeup under an overhead light**—it casts distorting shadows!

More Organizing Tips:

• Keep daily vitamins, any daily medicines in another bag or straw basket. Easy to get at!

• Keep teeth-care items (floss, mouthwash, etc.) in another—nail-care items in another.

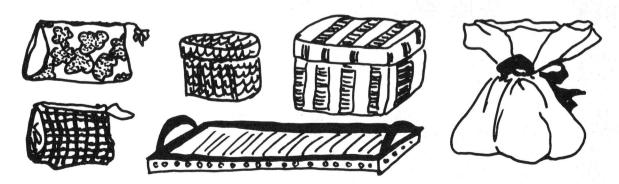

48

Makeup Checklist—Day

Foundation

Cover stick (concealer)

Small wedge-shaped silk sponges to apply foundation, cream blush, and for final after-powder makeup setting

Cotton swabs (for cleaning off mascara specks, etc.)

Eye cup (to hold water for cleanups!)

Eyelash curler

Lipbrush

Eyedrops (to wet down mascara, etc., instead of brush-in-mouth technique!)

Sharpener for pencils

Eyebrow/lash/brush/comb

Brushes:

• Eye makeup brushes (2)

• Thin one for concealer (to get in corners under eye!)

• Cheek color brushes (2)

• One for finishing powder (soft and full to dust all over face!)

Mascara (dark brown)

Loose transparent powder

Two lipglosses: one clear, one colored

Lipliner pencil (skin-colored!)

Eyeliner pencil: a soft smoke-colored one

Eyeshadow: one deep, smokey brown or dark taupe

Cheek color: tawny or burnt rose

One lip color: tawny or burnt rose

Tip: For more organization ease, (1) keep *makeup tools* (brushes, sharpeners, etc.) *in one container*; (2) *keep makeup in another*. (3) *Keep special evening makeup in another.*

Evening Makeup Checklist

Gold eyeshadow (powder) + one brush for applying to eye area + one thicker brush for dusting gold on face, cheeks, etc.

Eyeshadow—dark shadow-tone eyeshadow: dark olive black-green or dark smoke gray or dark browny taupe

Charcoal eyeliner pencil

Charcoal mascara

Cheek color—one rosy or clear red cheek color

Extra lip colors—orangey reds (for fluorescent light . . . museum openings, theatre, etc.) Rosy reds for candlelight . . . restaurant dinners, dark night-cluby places, etc.)

Skin Care Checklist

Eye cream

Moisturizer (day)

Night cream

Skin cleanser (makeup remover)

Eye makeup remover

Skin toner

Cleansing mask

Cotton balls

Tweezers

Magnifying mirror

Blemish medicine if you use one

Hair band or cotton scarf (to keep hair cleanly off face)

Nail Care Checklist

Emery boards

Orange stick

Pumice stone (one smooth one for fingers, one for feet!)

Cuticle cream

Hand cream

Polish remover

Cotton

Cuticle clippers

Clear polish

Base coat

one or two most-used-color polishes (a pale tone for day, a scarlet/bordeaux for night and toes!)

White stick (for under nails when wearing clear polish)

Small scissors

Cotton swabs (for cleaning under nails)

A small bottle of peroxide (for stubborn nail stains)

Hair Checklist

Brush (one with bristles bedded in a rubber base!)

Comb

Wide-tooth comb (for wet hair)

Covered rubber bands

Hairpins

Hair combs, barettes, etc.

Lengths of ribbon—black satin, black grosgrain, leather cord (to tie up or tie back hair)

Hair bands (tortoise, plastic, etc.)

Special Checklist for "Working Women"

For midday and end-of-day repairs—for the last-minute office-to-dinner evening!
In your desk keep a series of pretty cotton bags:

A makeup survival bag:

Magnifying mirror

Tweezers

Tissues

Small bottle of moisturizer

Small bottle of skin toner (for when you *can't* redo all your face!)

Foundation/sponges

Loose powder/brush

Blush/brush

Eye shadow/brush (dark brown!)

Eyeliner pencil—dark brown or taupe

Lipstick

Lipgloss—clear

Mascara (brown)

Spray can of mineral water (refreshes—doesn't remove makeup!)

Fragrance

Hair survival bag:

Brush

Comb

Small hairspray and cotton (to slick down ends). *Remember: Always apply spray by spraying onto cotton* and "dusting" over hair— you'll find it's less damaging than spraying directly on hair!

Some lengths of black and deep tones of satin ribbon

Pairs of combs (tortoise, gold)

Covered rubber bands

A small set of hot curlers to "re-zip" hair

Nail repair bag:

Remover/cotton

Base

Polish: clear plus "your color"—don't forget toes!

Emery boards

Hand cream

In another bag: soap, liquid makeup remover, toothbrush and toothpaste, breath freshener, Band-Aids. A small towel! **In another bag:** sewing kit, lint remover, extra pair of pantyhose, a change of underwear. (A fresh bra and panties—if you've time—can make you feel as if you had had time to go home and change for the evening!)
If you often do office-to-restaurant evenings, have a small evening bag—a "neutral" peanut kid or dark bordeaux kid (a "neutral" to what you might wear during the day) and even a pair of bare neutral-toned leather high-heeled sandals.

• A.M. and P.M.: Cleanse, tone, nourish skin

• A.M. and P.M.: Cream on hands and cuticles

• A.M. **or** P.M.: Wash and condition hair (one shampooing)

• Same time daily: Check weight (key to keeping track of weight gain!) It makes dieting almost unnecessary!

• Exercise: ten minutes A.M. and P.M. (Stretches—A.M. and Aerobics—P.M. to energize!)

• A.M. Vitamins

Weekly Beauty/Health Routines

• Manicure/ pedicure

• Maintenance skin cleaning (professional is best, especially if you live in a city!)

• At least two group exercise (or yoga or dance) classes a week! A "group" means you work hardest and fully.

• If possible, have a therapeutic massage—especially if your work keeps you working on "nerves!"

Monthly

• Haircut or trim

• A penetrating conditioner on hair with heat cap.

• (Professional deep-skin cleaning. If you have problem skin, see a dermatologist! Don't rely on an esthetician!

• Check arms, legs and facial hair for bleaching, waxing.

Every Six Months:

Every six Months:
• Dentist

• Doctor—health check

Yearly:

• Clean out medicine cabinet. Out-of-date medicines can be useless—or dangerous!

• **Ideal rest-cure:** Try to get away to a health spa for one week of cleansing diet, body care, etc., or do it yourself.

• *Do it yourself spa*: Take a "vacation" alone with your favorite books, music, and a refrigerator of: fresh fruit, vegetables, water, white meat chicken, fresh (poached) fish. (1) Keep to 1,000 calories maximum a day. (Get a calorie counter!). (2) Drink tons of water! (3) Do a one-hour exercise tape religiously *daily*! See *bath section* for recipes for therapeutic baths. (4) Do facial steaming with herbs, skin cleansing masks; scrub body with a loofa in the shower to make body skin baby-new ... (5) Moisturize skin constantly. (6) Go to sleep with heavily moisturized hands and feet (warm petroleum jelly is fabulous) plus white cotton gloves and socks. Try warming all creams to help them penetrate deeper! (7) Give hair a treatment—a hair nourishing pack and heat cap (you'll find this really helps creams to penetrate hair)! (8) Wear no makeup!

10-MINUTE MAKEUP FOR DAY

Rule: You Should Never Be Able to Notice Your Makeup—Only its Effect!

Tips for modern, EASY attractive makeup

Application

1. As light a hand as possible.

Color

2. As naturally toned as possible! Go with your natural coloring—*don't* try to change it! If your skin is yellow (sallow), use a creamy, slightly yellow (rather than rosy) toned foundation. If you have freckles, don't try to cover them. If you have pale lips, don't try to enhance them by darkening . . . keep them pale!

How to Begin

• **Putting on makeup should be a pleasant ritual.** The TRICK: Have all your needs and tools organized. THEN RELAX. Remember, the goal of putting on makeup is to make you look even *more* attractive. **You must begin by feeling good.**

• Remember, "less is more!" You can always add. It's hard-to-impossible to remove excess makeup without beginning from scratch!

• Lay everything out on your little tray. Think of a doctor and his instruments! If you do this, the makeup ritual will take the *minimum time!*

• *Before* applying makeup, make sure skin surface is *cool.* Makeup goes on better and "settles" better this way.

TIP: *Never* try any new makeup, makeup color, or makeup trick just before you have to look wonderful! *Test anything new* when you have the time to experiment . . . Remember those rainy weekend afternoons.

TIP: Get in the habit of applying makeup products with applicators—*not fingers.* Brushes, sponges, cotton-tipped sticks, etc. This way makeup goes on better, lighter, cleaner!

• **Key Tip:** *Check out your makeup light.* Make sure it's even. Make sure it doesn't come from overhead or from one side. *To get the best day makeup light,* turn your back to a window. North light exposure is ideal! Face your mirror, which reflects the daylight!

This is the light in which you will be seen. *Best evening makeup light:* a theatrical makeup mirror with bulbs all around. Buy the kind with lights that adjust to different "atmospheres" — candlelight, etc.

Pre-Makeup

1. Use a scarf or makeup band to get your hair off your face.

2. Always begin makeup with a thoroughly cleansed face.

3. *Moisturizer* preparation: *Always* put moisturizer on skin before foundation! **Trick:** Pour a little moisturizer onto back of your nonworking hand. Dot with tips of fingers of working hand on face: forehead, cheeks, the tiniest bit on chin, neck. *Skip your nose—* it's the oiliest part! Smooth moisturizer in gently. Blot with tissue to remove any excess. Rub leftover amount on nonworking hand into hands, elbows, knees, etc. . . . economy!

• **CONCEALER** *Covering step* (to mask dark circles, mouth creases, etc.) *Rule:* Light areas "move forward." Dark areas recede. Therefore, to lift areas "out of shadows," use *a concealer* (one tone lighter than foundation!) to lighten. Or use a *tone of foundation lighter than your all-over foundation*. Use on under-eye circles, recessed corners of mouth, deep laugh lines ... **never on raised areas** such as blemishes. It makes them stand out more!

Trick to apply: *Dot on* concealers using a *thin sable brush*. The brush distributes and blends into corners better than fingers and allows you to control the amount applied. Remember, you can always add more!

• FOUNDATION

Trick: Always *match foundation color to skin color of neck* (never to hands, as one is often prompted to do at makeup counters!). Hands are your *most* exposed skin; they never match face skin color! *If you match to your neck you don't risk a demarcation line where foundation stops* and your neck begins! **Foundation color rule:** a lighter tone of foundation is safer than darker! Always!

Trick to apply: Use back of hand pallette technique to apply. Pour a small amount of foundation onto back of non-working hand. Dot onto face: forehead, cheeks, next to nose, chin. Gently blend out towards hairline and out onto ears. You don't want light ears gleaming out! With what's *left* on fingertips blend onto neck—the bare minimum of foundation for a "hint" only, to even everything out.

Trick for extra natural foundation: *Blend* again with a water-dampened silk sponge. *This is the key to perfect, sheer, natural-looking foundation cover.* It *sets the foundation* and makes it smooth and extra transparent—natural! Blot gently with a tissue. *The secret to great natural makeup is blotting!* It sets each layer and removes any excess. Important: When applying foundation over areas masked with concealer, always pat gently or you will remove the covering layer!

Tip: If your skin is *oily*, use a *water-based* foundation; if *dry*, a moisturizing foundation.

• BLUSH

• General rule: Use cream rouge for day. It's more natural-looking. Add powder rouge for night for a matte, more "made-up" look!

• For day: Keep blush color in rosy or warm coral-tawny tones. Save the raspberries and fuchsias for night.

• How to apply:

1. Find your cheekbones. Tap the tips of your fingers along them. This is where the blush goes.

2. Smile into a mirror. The "apples" of your cheeks are the place to begin, for a natural, healthy "glow" of blush.

• Dip middle finger into cream rouge. Rub thumb and middle finger together to even and thin the blush. This keeps you from winding up with a glob of color and the rubbing warms the cream and makes it blend easier!

• Blend blush by *patting*— never rubbing or dragging!— along cheekbones up into hairline. Finish with a dash onto earlobes. Otherwise ears stand out as "pale strangers!" BLEND *with a damp sponge* (a light *patting*) to set.

Trick: For more "healthy glow," add a touch of blush color high up on forehead at the corners and into hairline.

Where to apply blush if Your Face Is:

Round: Keep color on apples of cheek. *Do not* blend beyond apples onto cheekbone and to hairline. This way the color concentration is towards *center* of face. The sides of your face seem to recede!

Long: To add width, start blush beyond "apples" ... Keep it *only on cheekbone* with *concentration of color out toward hairline and ears*. The eye is drawn to the color at *sides* of face and *away* from center of face, thereby widening the effect!

Square (strong jaw): To soften the angular line, focus attention on your eyes. Concentrate the blush in a triangle on cheek just under the center of your eye. Begin blush application on cheekbone. The point of the triangle is directed toward the center of eye. Blend well so that there is no demarcation line. Remember to keep it all very subtle and light-handed! *Practice* for ease and for the best effect!

EYES

General Rule: For the most natural and effective eye makeup, think **Natural Shadow** Colors: browns, taupes, smoky grays, etc.

Beware of black. It can be very hard and harsh-looking. You must have an expert light hand to use black shadow effectively without a Theda Bara result! Practice at home when you have time if you want the effect of black shadow. Use very sparingly.

• LASHES

1. *If you curl your lashes*, do so *before* applying mascara. After mascara you risk breaking lash hairs!

2. *Mascara tips.* Use brown mascara for day, black at night. Apply only to *tips* of lashes. Important: *Keep mascara layers extra thin!* Three to four thin layers are better-looking, healthier for lashes, and infinitely more effective than one thick globby layer! Make sure each layer has time to dry before the next application. Work on the rest of eye

makeup in between applications to save time. Always mascara both top and bottom lashes—never one without the other!

TIP: After each layer dries, brush out lashes with a baby toothbrush or eyebrow brush to separate lashes and remove excess mascara.

Note: You can do the Mascara Step *before Covering Foundation Steps.* This eliminates any lash smudges on cheeks which could be hard to remove without removing foundation.

TRICK: To remove smudges, dip a cotton swab in water. Press on towel to remove excess water. *Dot* on skin gently to remove smudge. Don't rub!

TRICK: For too much mascara on lashes, wet a baby toothbrush. Brush out lashes with damp toothbrush.

Tip: If you have very light lashes, think about having them professionally tinted. In the long run it's better and easier than constant mascara-ing!

• EYE SHADOW

How to apply: Use powder eye shadow. It's easier to control, looks softer, more normal, and doesn't melt into lid creases.

1. Blot lids. They must be free of oil. Trick: Pat lids gently with foundation sponge to leave just a hint of matte base. This helps keep shadow "smooth."

2. With soft shadowing brush take up color—a dark

milk chocolate brown or taupy gray for day! **Rule:** The best eye shadow colors are the same colors and tones of natural shadows . . . smoke tones! Flick out excess eye shadow powder on brush, tapping as you would a cigarette.

• Begin application in the outside corner of eye where lids meet. This is where the concentration of color will be. Gently trace the brush up into crease of eyelid and onto the underside of eyebone to just-beyond-center-of eye (towards nose). Then trace the brush along the *base* of your lashes, upper lid, to just-beyond-center-of eye, towards nose. Next, trace the brush along base of lashes, lower lid, to the same spot, just-beyond-center-of eye, towards nose. You have made a wide triangle.

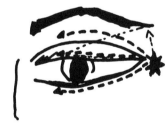

• *Begin now to intensify and diffuse* the shadow with the brush (re-dipped and flicked out). Begin at starting spot (outside corner where lids meet) and follow the original path until you have the intensity of color that you want. Work brush in a *slightly* upward movement toward eyebone and then around and

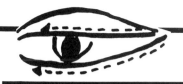

down toward lid center. You are defining a triangle, the base of which is at outside of eye to bone (parallel to temples), the point of which is center eye toward lash base of upper lid.

• Keep blending, adding a *little* color at a time. Remember, *color concentration is at outside corner* . . . as you move in toward nose it becomes less and less to nothing! As you move up toward eyebone it becomes less and less to nothing.

• **Eye Shadow Tips**

Key: The under-lash shadow line must be kept close to the *root* of lower lid lashes. If it extends too low below the lid, you create a no-sleep-for-days circles under your eyes effect.

• *Do not* extend the lash rimming lines to the *inside* corners of eyes. This tends to "close" the eye and makes it look smaller.

To emphasize eye.

With a soft brown or taupe *pencil*, gently overtrace shadow line along lash roots, top and bottom lid, to just beyond center of eye toward nose (*very, very* close to root of lashes!).

• Diffuse and blend with a cotton swab. First run the swab in *toward the nose*. Then out *toward temples*, stopping where eyelids meet.

Important: (1) Smudge, do not *line*! (2) Work as close to lash *roots* as possible!

Where/How to Apply Shadow If You Have

A long face: Blend eye shadow straight across lid toward temples to create horizontal effect.

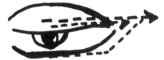

A round face: Run the shadow in more toward nose. Blend out and up toward the outside edges of forehead. Keep color concentration *toward* the center of eye—*not* at outside edge!

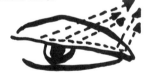

A square face: Angle a "triangle" of shadow up on lids toward forehead corners *away* from the temples and a "horizontal line!"

Shadow Tricks

If your eyes are spaced far apart. (1) **Do** concentrate shadow toward *inside* corners of eyes, at nose. This gives the illusion of bringing them in! (2) Apply mascara more heavily at inner lashes top and bottom and barely nothing at outside lashes!

If your eyes bulge: Be sure

to line lower lid with shadow. Dark shadows recede! "Smoke" the entire upper lid with brown. Again, dark shadows recede! *Center the mascara application at top and bottom of lashes* in the middle of eyes—not at the sides of lashes!

If your eyes are too close together: Accent *outside* corners of eyes. Do *not* extend shadow further in (toward nose) than midcenter of eye. Apply mascara more heavily at *outside* lashes top and bottom and barely *nothing* from the center of the eye in!

If your eyes are deep-set: Use brown shadow only along lash *roots*, top and bottom. Extend and blend the line up and out at the point where the upper and lower lashes meet. Highlight! Use a *very light* tone and taupe or pale brown (beige) shadow on the lid and onto the browbone to create the effect of your eyes coming forward. Remember the rule: Light areas move forward. Run a diffused line of dark brown shadow in the eyelid crease from the center of the lid and out. Blend it into the two lashliner lines (up and out). Apply mascara *only* on outer lashes top and bottom.

General Note on "Highlighters"

Any pale to white to silver-toned shadow-powders and creams are considered highlighters. The safest way to "highlight" until you are an expert is with a *paler tone of your eye shadow color* (with brown shadows, a pale taupe—with grays, a pale gray, etc.). *Do not* try silver, gold, pink, etc., until you really know what what you are doing.

Remember: Light areas are emphasized—dark areas recede. White and silver highlighters are like lightbulbs . . . The area where you put them will stand out. Study your face. **Touch it**. Touch the bones, the way the muscles move. Practice! If you have a prominent browbone *do not* apply highlighter to it. It will only become more prominent. If you want to accent your cheekbones (especially nice at night!), dot some highlighter high on the bone and out towards temples. It gives a lift to your face!

Brows

Tip: Brows should be ideally one to two shades lighter than your hair! Have them bleached professionally once to see the effect. It immediately softens your face—great "age" trick!

• How to Proportion Brows

1. Brush out brows with a brow brush/comb, first toward nose (against the growth) and then up and out toward temples (with the growth).

2. Use a pencil as a measure.

3. Place pencil vertically on face, one end at *beginning* of brow. This point should line up with inner corner of eye and base of nose. If necessary *add* more brow with a pencil with *light* feather strokes—keep the color of the pencil the color of your eyebrow—or tweeze out excess hairs.

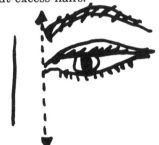

4. Then, place pencil diagonally, one end at outer base of nose, the other lining up with *outer* corner of *eye*. Lengthen the brow if necessary with light, short feather strokes to reach this point. Brow should line up with outer corner of eye!

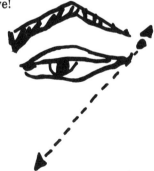

Tip for a natural un-makeup-y eyebrow. Add pencil color a *little at a time*—you can always add more! As you pencil, keep brushing brows out to blend color and study the line. Walk away and then look at brows again in a full-length mirror. This is a good proportion test. "Finish" face before doing mouth.

Powder

Loose translucent powder is key to a beautifully finished and natural makeup! Apply powder with cotton balls. You then throw them away—more sanitary than a puff!

How to powder:

Dip cotton ball in powder. Shake out cotton to remove excess. Gently *dab* face. "Press, release . . . press, release" is the motion. *Never* drag puff on face, as it removes the underlayers of foundation and color. *Do not powder lips—it makes lip color cake!* Then, blend powder with a wide-tipped sable brush, gently dusting face all over. Be sure to dust over eyelids. This helps tone down and set eye makeup!

Tip: For an *unpowdery* and extra-translucent look: *set the powder*. Dip a clean cotton ball in water. Wring out well. Then gently press it all over face *except your nose*, as it is the first spot to get shiny! This fixes the powder, removes any excess, and makes your skin look beautifully fragile and glowing.

Mouth

How to line your lips:

1. For the most natural un-makeup-looking mouth: Use a pencil that is *lip skin color*.

Never use a lipstick color as a pencil because it is too harsh a line!

2. Trace pencil gently and lightly along the natural lipline at the bow of upper lips only, from one side of bow to the other. Then make a bit of a line just under the lower lip at the center of lip only. Blend the lines with a fingertip out toward corners of lips.

Trick for thick lips: Follow the same directions but trace the line just inside the natural lip line. Use a paler rather than strong lip color afterwards. Pale means toward skin tone—not whitened!

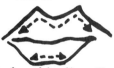

Trick for thin lips: Run the line *outside* your natural lipline. Fill the space between lip and traced line with a lipbrush dipped in a lip color that is ONE SHADE DARKER than your final lip color. Blot. Then apply final lip color, but only up to natural lipline—not beyond. A thin layer of powder over all blends and softens lines and sets the colors.

HOW TO APPLY LIP COLOR:

3. AFTER LIPLINER IS BLENDED, APPLY LIP COLOR WITH A *BRUSH*.
• Begin in the middle of lips at center, near inside of mouth. This should be your point of heaviest color concentration.
• Blend out and up and out and down toward lip edges, but never all the way to edge.
• Apply a thin layer of gloss over it all. This gloss layer blends and diffuses lip color toward edges in a natural way. Lips never "run" with color!

Lipstick Color Trick: Keep cheeks and lips in same color range! This looks most natural. For example: burgundy mouth/rose cheeks (not peach; it's too yellow a tone!), bronze cheeks/apricot mouth (rose or burgundy is too blue a tone).

LIP TIPS

1. Use a brush! You can control the color, and it makes a neater, more natural, and *smoother* mouth.

2. Bright scarlet lip color brings out the yellow in teeth. Watch out! Paler apricot, rose, tawny tones are easiest to live with, especially during the *day*!

3. Don't powder lips—It makes lip color cake.

4. If lips become cracked, chapped:
• Use medicated lip cream, anti-chap creams, etc.
• Don't lick lips—especially drying in sun and cold!

• Apply a thin layer of gloss or moisturizer *before* lip color.
• Use an extra *thin* layer of color. Too much color accentuates cracks!

Time: Day Makeup—maximum fifteen minutes
Practice!
You should be able to get day makeup routine down to *ten minutes*!

If You Wear Glasses

• Watch out for *too* much eye and cheek makeup! Prescription lenses tend to magnify eyes, make them look larger, and *intensify* the effect of makeup. Adjust!
• Keep to warm shadow tones on eyes: honeys, bronzes, etc.
• Oversized lenses will accentuate cheek color. Adjust.
• Tip: Stick to classic frame shapes and classic frame colors. Rounded, ovaled shapes rather than square or wing-shaped. Clear, pale or tortoise-toned frames (from pale amber to rich dark brown) are best for day. Black frames are hard to wear, literally! They sharpen and "close in" face. If you choose them, try tinting lenses a shade or two darker than clear to keep the contrast from frame to lense less acute.

Rule: Overly tricky and "fashiony" glasses can be amusing, but you must be sure that you *want* to be amusing...and that you can carry them off without looking silly or odd!

TWENTY-FOUR WAYS TO

The Key Classic Shapes

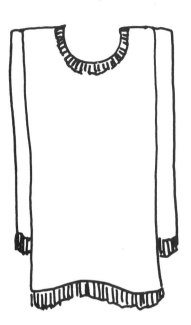

Crewneck

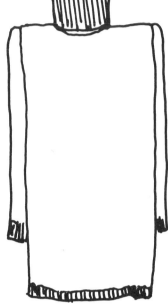

Turtleneck

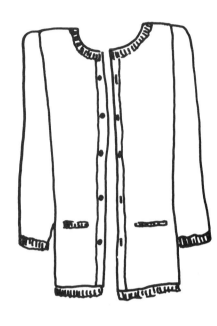

Cardigan

When You Buy Sweaters

• Buy the best possible yarn. *Cashmere is ideal. Angora/lambswool* is often so well combined it is almost as soft as cashmere! *Soft wool.*

• Stay away from anything too stiff or too limp, too fancy (as lacy or multi-stitched), *too heavy!* Buy the most classic unribbed knitstitch possible.

• *Buy in sets*: a cardigan, its crewneck, and even its turtleneck if it's the shape for you. The trick here is to build a collection you will be able to add

to—*and use*—season after season, year after year. Some designers often do an evening sweater version as part of their sweater collections. . . . If you find a strapless, halter or camisole sweater that also works in, buy it! It is a valuable find for dozens of late-day looks!

Note: For warm climates look for cotton-knit sweaters or cotton/rayon, silk or silk and cashmere combinations. Follow the same ground rules!

• If you live in the country, add Shetland and Irish knit to your collection.

Shape Recommendations

• For turtleneck substitute loose, short cowlneck (it sits *away* from neck) if you have a short neck, a too-round face, or double chin problem. It gives a sense of more length as it shows skin, and isn't binding!

• The ideal cardigan to really "perform" in your life is one that falls straight from shoulder to hem including ribbing, as opposed to those with ribbing that pulls in. A straight cardigan works as a "jacket" and can be made to look late-day!

WEAR A SWEATER

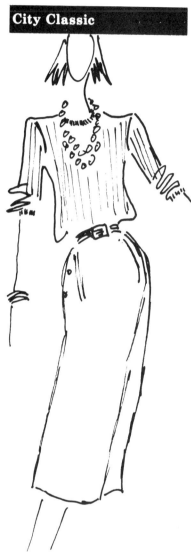

• Crewnecked sweater, *matching* narrow easy skirt or pant—like a painter's canvas! Take a beige sweater, beige wrap skirt (or gray or navy or taupe); add a pretty belt. Tone your shoes and stockings. You can then put almost anything over: a mini-check tweed jacket in tones of brown to beige, a navy blazer, a quilted olive cotton cardigan jacket, a navy jersey unlined 7/8 coat, a fur, a raincoat...even a brown velvet cardigan!

Trick: Blouse and belt the sweater slightly at waist for softness. Keep the belt on the narrow side and always *toned* to the color of the skirt and sweater for one long unbroken line.

Note: With grays or navy, shades of brown leather count in the "toning" category. You do *not* have to match belt exactly to skirt and sweater! Try a deep-colored belt and shoe (bordeaux leather belt, bordeaux leather shoe) if you are long and slim enough to break the line! Always add pretty jewelry (some gold bracelets, a necklace of gold and carnelian or tiger-eye beads) for finish.

• If you have big hips, do *not* belt the sweater. Think tunic! Make sure the sweater falls straight and smooth and does not cling. **Always match skirt and sweater.**

Note: With the city-*trouser* version of this look (trouser and heeled or flat shoe) always try to *match* stocking or *sock* to shoe to give the "one-color" effect of a boot (one continuous line). To see a flash of skin between trouser and shoe is an instant leg shortener!

• A pretty trick: If you've the neck length, stand the notched collar of the blouse up and wrap it around your neck one point over the other. Pin it closed with a narrow gold stick pin or gold safety pin. The effect: a silk turtleneck!

• Be sure to turn blouse cuffs over sweater cuffs for a pretty touch of "color and finish."

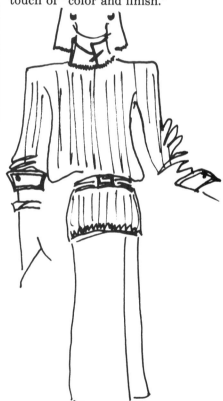

• If your sweater and bottom tone well and you have no hip problems, wear sweater *over*

TWENTY-FOUR WAYS TO WEAR A——

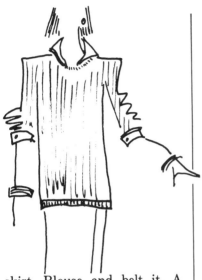

skirt. Blouse and belt it. A Look: a pale rose silky blouse under a gray sweater, over a gray flannel wrap skirt; pigskin belt with brass buckle, pigskin-toned (peanut) leather day pump, tan-toned stockings; dark brass and wood bangles. Or wear the collar of blouse open (especially if you need neck length). Stand it up a bit in back. Fill the neckline with some pretty gold beads and chains or nothing but skin. For finish be sure to add a flash of earrings!

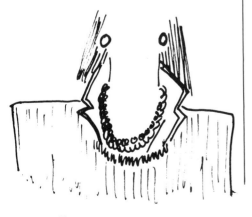

Country Version

• A cream-silk shirt under a pale blue Shetland pullover, tan corduroy jeans, peanut loafers and—if your legs are long enough—pale blue socks! A classic country finish: Your old Harris tweed hacking jacket, still perfect after five years!

Tip: If this is your life-style, look for hacking jackets in riding shops. They are timeless, classicly shaped, *and* of the best cloth.

Instant easy country/resort look

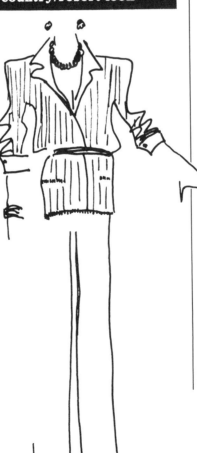

• White blouse/white cotton *jeans* (or trousers), navy cardigan over, belted in hemp rope. Be sure to turn the blouse cuffs up or over sweater for dash! Add white canvas espadrilles or flat red kid sandals, some pretty pale wood or ivory beads, bracelets, and you are set for lunch or drinks at a private home or dinner at a seaside restaurant.

NOTE: How to wear cardigan: try buttoning it only at waist, blousing slightly, belting.

• If you have big hips, match the cardigan to skirt or trouser. Wear another color blouse for a dash. Do *not* belt cardigan! Wear loose and open as you would a "cardigan jacket."

• Country *winter* version: peanut corduroy jeans (or skirt), cream shirt, vicuña-colored cardigan, belted in peanut and brass-edged leather. Add mahogany-colored boots or vicuña woolly tights and moccasins.

Take a cowl or turtleneck sweater and a skirt (or trouser). Match or tone them closely

• Add a pretty clip to the edge of turtleneck near the collarbone. For more neck, wear a small cowl sweater—it's loose at neck—and pull one side of the cowl asymmetrically askew with a pretty clip. This shows

SWEATER

even more skin and *makes for neck length*! Example: Brown turtleneck, brown skirt—add dark oxblood belt—brown toned legs—same-toned brown leather shoes—some earrings,

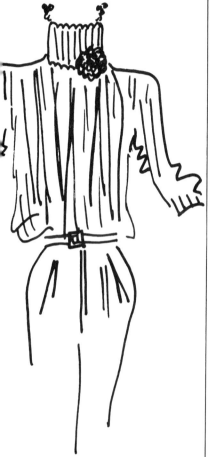

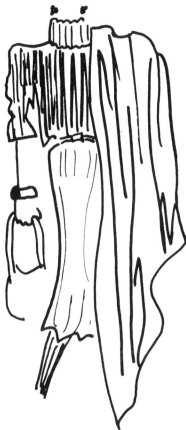

and you have another great work/town look! For dash, fling a thin bordeaux wool shawl over your shoulders—or short cardigan jacket of camel-and-brown tweed or dark brown velvet (yes, for day!)—or your tan poplin trenchcoat!

Version 2—matching turtleneck (or cowl) and skirt and a cardigan of a second color.

• Gray turtleneck, gray flannel skirt. Over it, a vicuña-colored (or bordeaux or black) cardigan belted in pigskin or walnut

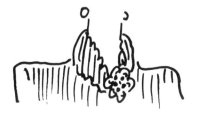

leather, shoe and stocking toned together and toned to belt color. Close cardigan at waist only, blouse, and then belt.

• *Remember*: If you have big hips or want more body-leg length, *match cardigan to skirt*. Then belt or wear cardigan loose, depending on how skinny you need to look

• *Trick for dash*: Turn turtleneck cuff over cardigan cuff—a nice finish of another color cuff!

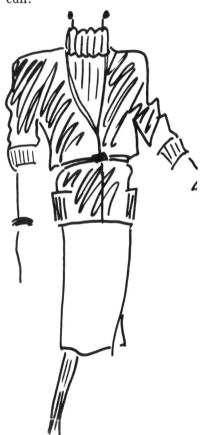

TWENTY-FOUR WAYS TO WEAR A——

• Start with cream sweater (turtleneck or crew). Add cream wool trousers, gold belt, gold sandals, wonderful gold with-a-touch-of-sparkle earrings, some gold beads at neck if you choose a crewneck sweater. Throw a pale peach soft wool shawl over one shoulder. Or do an all-black or all-navy version, add a scarlet shawl, short fur jacket, or quilted velvet ¾ *cardigan jacket* in a shade of cobalt blue. Do bronze or black satin belt and sandals instead of all gold. Add black onyx.

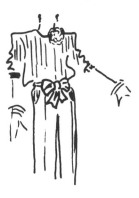

• For a bit of Evening Charm, pin a small gardenia or camellia to the sweater at the curve of the neck at collarbone.

• The trick: The addition of the gold or satin belt and sandals *plus* perfect hair, makeup, hands and feet, *plus* pretty jewelry equals a great-looking evening turnout for dinner, theatre, etc.!

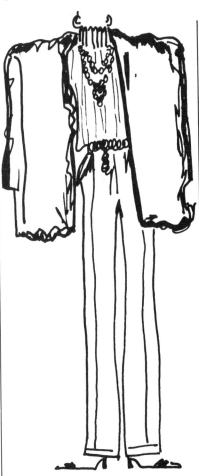

Chic at-home or to-dinner-at-friend's look:

• A black crewneck pullover plus long, slim, *soft* black silky, jersey, or velvet skirt. The trick: A skirt that is slim, soft, and easy—not a stiff "hostessy" skirt! Add evening sandals, glittery bracelets and earrings. You can do the gold belt/gold sandals here, too! Or, wear the sweater pulled smooth and unbelted, add color! Green or scarlet satin evening sandals, bracelets made of emerald-colored stones and gold and maybe one sliver of black lacquer.

For theatre/restaurants

• Cream sweater plus cream *short* silky or *soft* jersey skirt. Soft and silky is key—not hard or stiff! A slightly shirred-at-

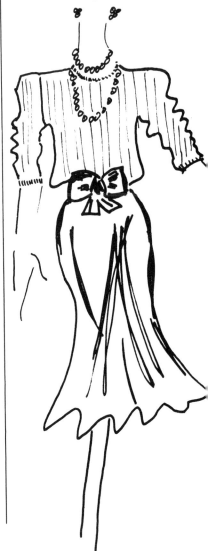

SWEATER

waist wrapskirt in jersey is pretty, attractive. You can do the same sweater and skirt in navy or black, add gold at waist and feet. Or tie a black satin ribbon bow at waist, wear beautifully shaped black satin pumps and sheer black stockings. Or for fun, try a *dark* cobalt blue satin ribbon at waist with black satin shoes and

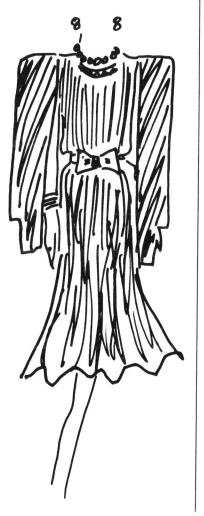

black stockings. Ribbon note: make sure you use pure *silk* satin ribbon to tie waists. It is expensive but worth the investment since they last. The less expensive qualities never look right! **For finish** add a black velvet jacket for the dark versions, a pale-toned shawl or jacket for cream or pale version, or throw the pullover's matching cardigan sweater over your shoulders for a perfect warmer-weather cover! Try a black crewneck sweater, black silky skirt, plus red cardigan sweater—**Great Dashing Look** with black satin shoe and evening bag and black sheer stockings.

Evening

• Take a cardigan sweater, skirt or trouser. Match cardigan to bottom (trouser or skirt). Add a **bare** halter, camisole, or strapless top—one in silk or satin that shows skin or a sweater knit. Black cardigan, black gabardine trousers, cream silk camisole. Belt all in black or red satin or gold kid. Add evening sandals, pretty jewels, **perfect makeup**. Another Look: try cardigan worn open over skirt and *belted* over a pretty print silk shirt. Or do the same over *matching* silky pajamas or gray flannel trousers. Add pretty shoes and jewelry, you have another easy evening look!

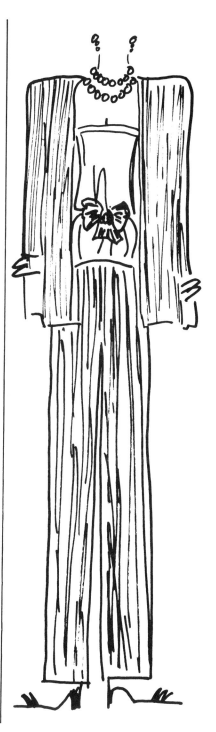

TWENTY-FOUR WAYS TO WEAR A——

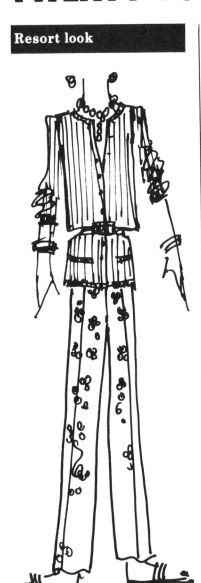

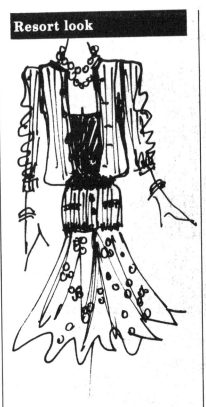

flower where the unbuttoning stops—a gardenia, camellia, small white orchid—and pret-

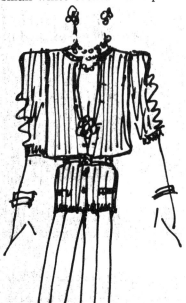

• White cardigan—opened as far as you dare—belted in gold over printed white-and-pale-blue tiny-flowered silky trousers. Add gold sandals, a lot of ivory-toned beads, gold earrings.

• For a really smashing resort look, try white cardigan belted in gold over white ground tiny multicolored flowered silky **skirt**. Wear bare camisole (to match color of one of the skirt print colors)—under cardigan. Add flat gold sandals.

At-home or dinner/ winter

• Wear either a pale blue or the palest pink cardigan unbuttoned low to show skin, over gray flannel trousers. Belt cardigan in gold kid or tie with a pale gray satin ribbon bowed at waist for an elegant and sophisticated effect. Add a fresh

ty bracelets. If it's your at-home dinner, wear flat ballet slippers in pink kid or flat pale rose satin sandals. If you're going out you'll want a dressier look. Wear gold kid sandals with heels or gray satin ones trimmed elegantly in gold.

Cardigan sweater and silk trousers

• A red cardigan knotted at the waist (as one would knot a shirt) over black silk trousers (*or* over a floaty, silky skirt). Wear over nothing but skin or slide a thin black strapless camisole under the cardigan. Add *lots* of gold jewelry. Wear flat black ballet slippers for at-home dinner; black- or red-

SWEATER

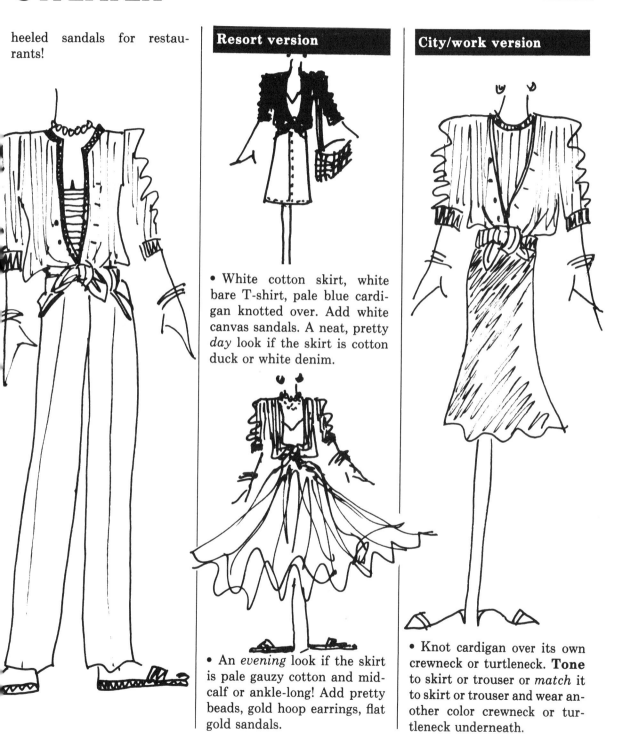

heeled sandals for restaurants!

• White cotton skirt, white bare T-shirt, pale blue cardigan knotted over. Add white canvas sandals. A neat, pretty *day* look if the skirt is cotton duck or white denim.

• An *evening* look if the skirt is pale gauzy cotton and midcalf or ankle-long! Add pretty beads, gold hoop earrings, flat gold sandals.

• Knot cardigan over its own crewneck or turtleneck. **Tone** to skirt or trouser or *match* it to skirt or trouser and wear another color crewneck or turtleneck underneath.

TWENTY-FOUR WAYS TO WEAR A——

• Red sweater under brown cardigan. Brown corduroy skirt, brown shoes and toned stockings.

• Beige turtleneck, beige cardigan, gray flannel trousers, walnut-heeled loafers, walnut leather shoulderbag, plus your favorite day jewelry.

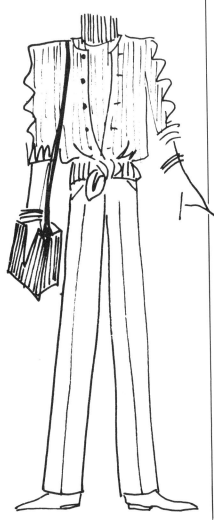

Instant suit look

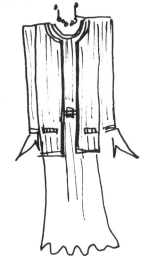

• *Cardigan and matching crewneck plus matching* soft *jersey skirt.* This is the moment when buying pieces that all tone together pays off. Add: pretty leather pumps, stockings toned to shoes, your best day gold jewelry (some chains at neck, small gold earrings). Add a leather envelope bag and you are turned out perfectly for a conference lunch, or a job interview—anywhere you want to look conservative and well-dressed. Add a short fur jacket, raincoat, or tweed ⅞ cardigan coat, depending on your basic wardrobe and the weather!

For dash—the double cardigan

• Try knotting a second cardigan in a dashing color over your shoulders when you wear

a cardigan with its matching crewneck or turtleneck (sweater set) **toned** to your skirt or trouser. For example: vicuña cardigan and crew, vicuña corduroy skirt, plus a scarlet cardigan around shoulders. This is especially handy if the two cardigans are the same shape.

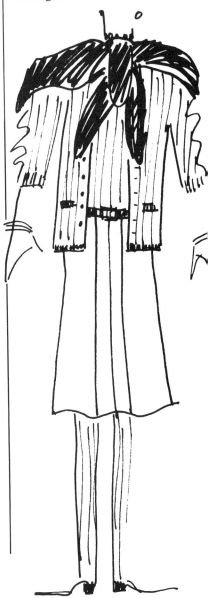

SWEATER

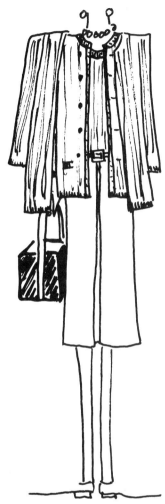

The red *looks* terrific (like a muffler shawl), and when it becomes cool slip it on. Remember, this takes a bit of wearing. If you aren't totally comfortable doing it, don't try it; otherwise you risk looking "unsure."

• Try a simpler version: a red cardigan knotted over shoulders with only the vicuña crewneck and matching vicuña cor-

duroy skirt. This way, the red one still can perform as a separate jacket and never be cumbersome. Note: *you are using color as an accessory*—the red cardigan is not only functional but the color red is as important as an arm of bracelets!

The cardigan as evening jacket

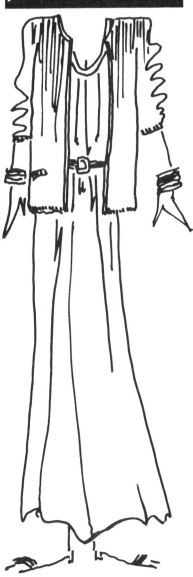

• Wear a cardigan sweater over a long jersey or sweatery tube of an evening dress: i.e., a black bare jersey dress with an emerald or claret-red cardigan sweater. Add a sliver of a gold belt and jewelry.

• Note: When doing any sweater look, remember always to keep the *oversweater lighter than underneath* tones to achieve the longest, skinniest look—if that's what you are after. *For example*: In the summer versions of navy sweater over white, substitute a white sweater or *pale* blue or pale cream if you need length for your body proportion.

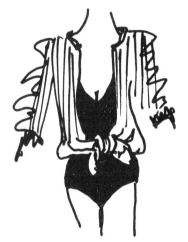

Beach sweater

• A sweater is a pretty bathing suit cover! Example: Pale pink cardigan knotted over a white maillot. Fabulous when you are a bit tan and there is a chill off the water!

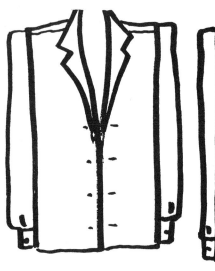

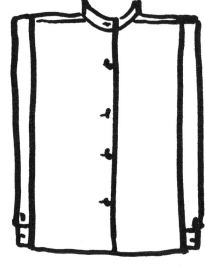

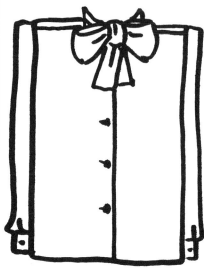

Notched-collar classic shirt

Collarband shirt

Ascot blouse

RECOMMENDATIONS

• The most versatile and *flattering* is a knotched-collared shirt/blouse *without* a collar stand. It is softer!

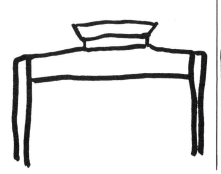

• Look for collars and cuffs *without* stiffening in lining. They are softer, more feminine, and you can do more "tricks" with them!

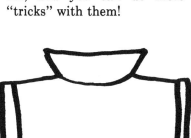

• The softer the fabric, the more versatile. Silk or silk-blend is best . . . soft cotton also. However, cotton *cannot* do evening duty except at times in summer! The ideal is to collect both. Begin building a shirt/blouse wardrobe.

• Look for blouses/shirts with straight bottoms rather than rounded bottoms.

You can then wear them both in and out.

• **Solid colors are most**

versatile. That does not mean a pretty stripe or check shouldn't be in one's collection. They add charm and diversion *but* the **solid tones do the hard work!**

• The less constructed the shirt, the more versatile—straight body as opposed to fitted, no pockets or only a *simple* breast pocket.

• Stay away from too much stitching, too many buttons (*especially* showy ones). Look for small four-hole pearl buttons matched to shirt fabric. **Remember, you are building a working collection.**

• Never bust darts in anything, especially a shirt!

Classic trim day look

• *Match blouse to skirt*: Pale beige silk blouse/beige wool wrap skirt. Add pigskin belt, shoes, and tan-toned stockings. Tie a small silk scarf at neck (perhaps a tan-and-cream print with a touch of peach stripe) or wear honey-colored carnelian or amber-toned beads with gold-toned bracelets.

• *A dashing touch*: Turn cuffs back instead of buttoning them—A more relaxed look, and bracelets show. A great turnout for office, school meeting, etc. *For cooler weather*: add another tone of jacket.

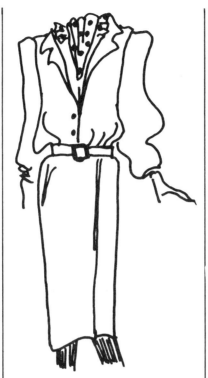

Since the underneath is all beige-toned, you could add a brown-and-cream tweed, tiny houndstooth or checked, or solid navy flannel jacket. Or wear a ¾ or ⅞ navy cardigan sweater thrown over your shoulders, or camel-colored ⅞ wool coat shaped like a Balmacaan raincoat!

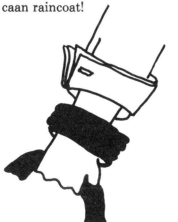

• Put a pretty color shirt on top to pull it together—a navy crewneck sweater tucked into a navy narrow (wrapped or front-pleated) skirt with a dark red or deep rusty-toned silky shirt on top.

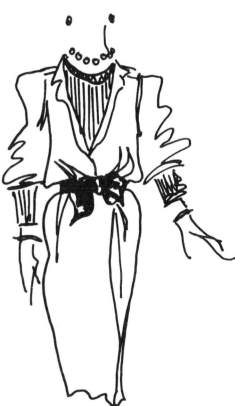

• *For dash*: Leave blouse unbuttoned and knot at waist. Roll and push up sleeves so that sweater cuffs show a bit. Add a pretty bracelet or two. For body length try navy-toned stockings and shoes.

TWENTY-FOUR WAYS TO WEAR A —

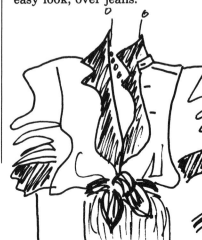

- *Variations*: The blouse could be (1) a "collarband shirt" worn over a cowl neck sweater perhaps, or (2) a *dark*-toned stripe (for instance, navy-red-black-and-cream narrow stripes) or (3) a tiny dot or checked silk.

length, tone the stocking and shoe to skirt (navy). Wear tan leather shoes and tan-toned stockings. Slip a tan leather belt around waist before tying shirt so that the belt shows a little and the tan tone of leg and shoe balance.

Double-blouses

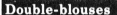

- *A cream blouse with a navy blouse on top*: If you are slim in hips, tuck both blouses into *navy* trousers or skirt or dark gray flannel trousers or skirt.

make a "*cuff*" of cream. Note: For maximum slimness wear darker-toned *over* lighter-toned blouse with the light tone *next to your skin* for an added skin-flattering bonus!

Trick: A pale color casts the most flattering light on your face! It also enables you to wear a slightly murky-toned color for an overshirt. For example, if you adore colors of the green or olive family and your skin has yellow tones, a cream or the palest pink *under*shirt gives your skin the most flattering lift, and then olive works beautifully.

Note: this look can also work with a *collarband blouse* worn over a *notched-collar* blouse. For country, try wearing these over a jeans skirt or, for a nice easy look, over jeans.

Same idea— different balance

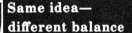

- Beige or red sweater, navy skirt, navy shirt to pull the look together. Again, for body

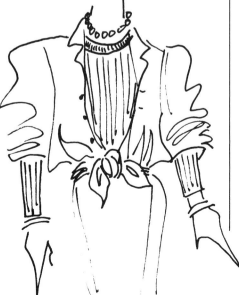

Belt in tan pigskin or tie the top blouse loosely at waist. The trick for double blouses is to wear the top one unbuttoned to the waist so the under one shows. Be sure to roll both the cream and navy sleeves together at the same time to

BLOUSE

• Tone an ascot blouse to skirt or trousers. Slide a knotched-collared blouse of another color over it all. For example, for evening: black ascot shirt, black pants, *red* overshirt. Add gold bracelets, black kid heeled sandals, a black-and-gold belt, gold earrings. A nice way to go to dinner at a restaurant.

• **Trick**: Wrap the ascot around and around and knot it in a **short**-knot instead of bowing it. Or pin ends closed with a pretty pin!

Another look: gray flannel skirt, gray ascot blouse, rust or dark rose overblouse. Belt it all in pigskin, add pigskin shoes, tan-toned stockings, gold earrings, a few bracelets. Super office look!

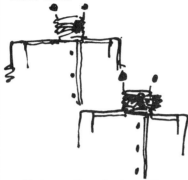

• *Hot weather look*: white ascot blouse, white cotton trousers. Add a raspberry overblouse, gold belt, gold flat sandals for summer dinner!

• *Romantic resort look*: a long or ankle-long white cotton-gauze, floaty *skirt*, white underblouse, pale cream overblouse. Be sure to open buttons as much as you dare, roll sleeves, belt in gold. Wear gold flat sandals. Tie your hair with a gold cord and add gold hoop earrings!

• *Remember*: The *ascot blouse* works only if you have neck length! If you are big-bosomed, if you have a short neck, a too-round face, or a double chin, do *not* wear this version. Do all the same looks with two notched-collared blouses or collarband/notched-collared versions. *These shapes show skin*; therefore they give the illusion of neck length!

More Ways to Wear a Blouse

• *Resort*—cream silk shirt open over cream cotton shorts. Slide a cream T-shirt under. Add red canvas belt, red kid sandals! Great way to look for lunch if you've got the legs! Otherwise do the same with a cream cotton skirt.

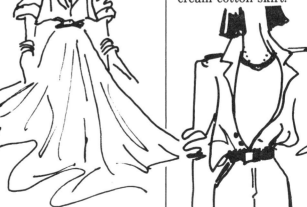

TWENTY-FOUR WAYS TO WEAR A ——

• *Resort:* the Biggest Shirt is the *best bathing suit cover*! Ideal: a large-sized man's silk shirt—*very* luxurious—or an oversized, well-washed, man's white cotton shirt! The key: the bigger the better! Roll the sleeves and wear loose.

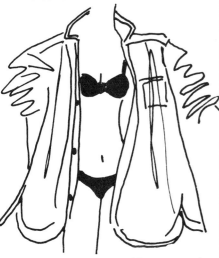

• *Resort: tie a blouse at the* waist over a bathing suit. Wrap a "sarong" over it as a

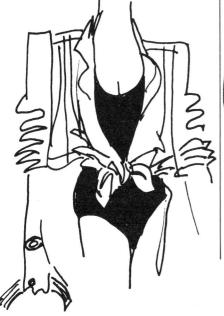

"skirt" for nifty instant go-to-lunch look! (See scarf section on how to tie a sarong.) Or, instead of sarong, wear a thin gauze ankle-long skirt, for example: yellow blouse, scarlet bathing suit, bright blue yellow-and-white-flowered sarong or cotton skirt.

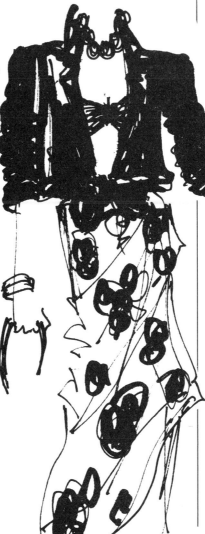

• ***Day/work:*** flannel, wool, tweed in gray, navy, beige, neutral tones.
• ***Resort/summer:*** hot sun colors—white, cream, sand colors in cotton, cotton gauze, cotton knit.
• Evening: Color and fabric are key. Black, jewel tones (burgundy, dark black-green), pale skin-beautiful colors (peach, pale pink), silk, velvet, thin jersey, thin crepe.

Quick great-looking instant evening

• Take a black velvet or jersey skirt or trouser. Add a black silk blouse. *Add—gold—*gold belt, gold or gold-and-black sandals, pretty gold and onyx jewelry. Or wear **black satin pumps,** black-toned stockings and a black *satin* belt. Add a lot of gold or gold-and-black bangles or cuffs! The key: pretty hair and *finished* makeup!

Tip: If you haven't the time for hair, *slick* it all back away from your face. (See hair section for "LOOKS.") Do a super-clean *finished* makeup. Wear your *prettiest* earrings to cast light to your face. You can then add a dark red satin cardigan, soft bordeaux paisley shawl, burgundy velvet jacket, or short fun jacket. You are beautifully turned out for theater, in any big city, anywhere. A great travel trick for Paris, London, Milan, etc.

BLOUSE

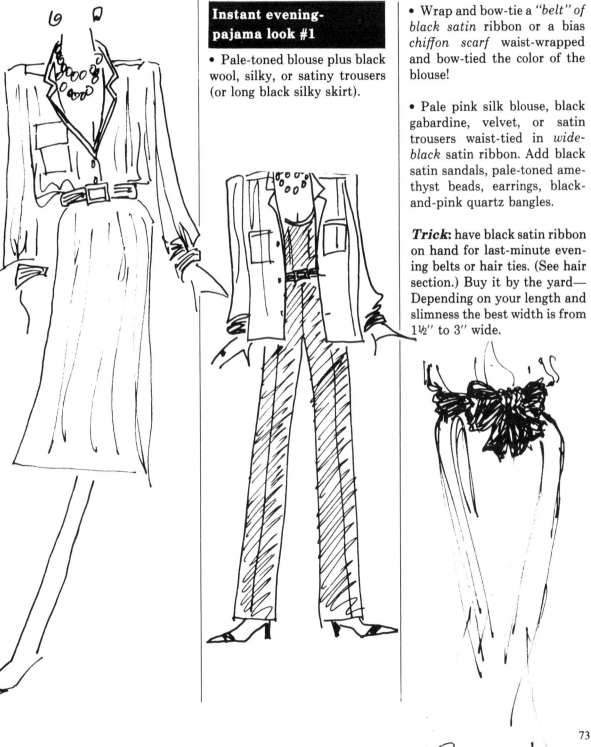

Instant evening-pajama look #1

• Pale-toned blouse plus black wool, silky, or satiny trousers (or long black silky skirt).

• Wrap and bow-tie a *"belt"* of *black satin* ribbon or a bias *chiffon scarf* waist-wrapped and bow-tied the color of the blouse!

• Pale pink silk blouse, black gabardine, velvet, or satin trousers waist-tied in *wide-black* satin ribbon. Add black satin sandals, pale-toned amethyst beads, earrings, black-and-pink quartz bangles.

Trick: have black satin ribbon on hand for last-minute evening belts or hair ties. (See hair section.) Buy it by the yard—Depending on your length and slimness the best width is from 1½" to 3" wide.

TWENTY-FOUR WAYS TO WEAR A —

• Pale pink silk blouse plus silk or jersey trousers or skirt in soft pale taupe. Wear blouse very open—push up and roll sleeves. Add some pale pink quartz and rock crystal necklaces and bracelets of quartz and gold; tuck a fresh flower in your hair. Tie a belt of long (multi-wrapped) bias of pale pink chiffon bowed at the waist. Wear pale pink satin ballet slipper or pale satin high-heeled sandals (depending on how tall you want to be). Or instead of chiffon scarf, belt in gold kid. Wear gold sandals and lots of *gold* jewelry.

Trick: for *soft* pajama look, keep the top tone *paler* than bottom. This gives a length illusion too! Example: Try cream blouse, pale bisque color or pale peach pants or long skirt with belt toned to the blouse, or one in gold or silver kid. Wear gold or silver sandals.

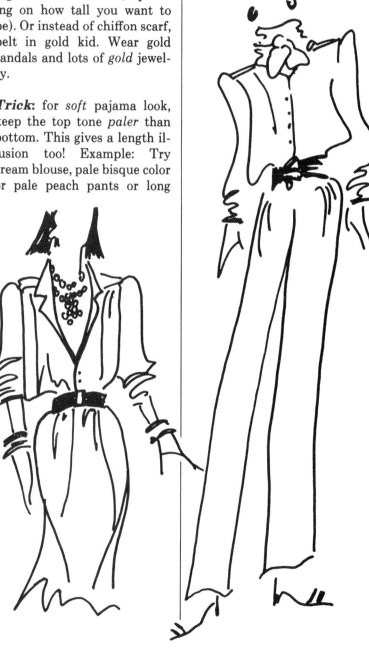

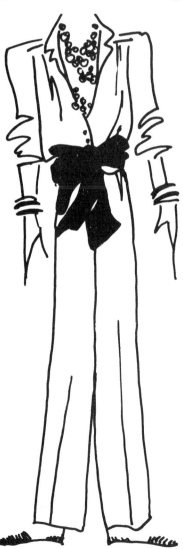

BLOUSE

• Pale gray ascot blouse knotted and wrapped high at the neck and held with a tiny fresh orchid or a pretty pin, gray flannel trousers, gold belt, and gold sandals. Add a short fur jacket, a cardigan jacket of bronze velvet, or a huge cashmere or soft wool shawl in cream or peach. A lovely way to look for an easy restaurant dinner or drinks-at-a-friend's!

Blouse: Instant jacket

• Slide a navy silk blouse over a bare bordeaux cotton knit dress. Terrific summer city look. *Now you see why simple straight body blouses are best!* Add wood bracelets, a belt of rope or tan leather, tan leather sandals, and straw shoulder bag.

• Or wear a bordeaux silk shirt as a *jacket* over navy or cream T-shirt, with bordeaux cotton trousers or skirt. Add tan leather belt, tan leather sandals, gold bangles, small gold hoop earrings or ear studs for great summer city look or *travel* look!

• White silk or thin cotton shirt as a *jacket* over: yellow T-shirt, yellow cotton pants or skirt. Add espadrilles or flat rope sandals and you have instant resort! This "jacket" is a great summer "cover" for overly air-conditioned shops, cinemas, etc.

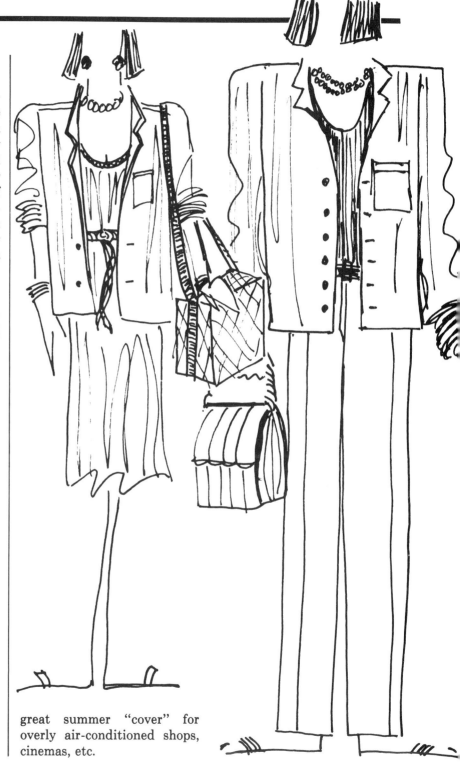

75

TWENTY-FOUR WAYS TO WEAR A——

Jacket for Summer Dinner

• Bare T-shirt top (black cotton knit), flower-printed silk or thin cotton skirt. For example, start with skirt colored black, red, and cream. Add red blouse as a *jacket*. Add red kid belt, red kid or black patent sandals, earrings, and bracelets.

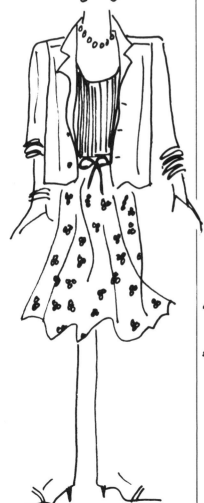

• The trick here is to make sure that T-top *and* blouse pick up some color of print of skirt. This way you pull it all together so that you get a *finished* look!

• This also could work with trousers: bare T-shirt top, *matching* thin cotton or silky trouser, a *pretty* color shirt as *jacket*. Add belt and sandals! The shirt could be a multi-stripe or print if other pieces are solid color *and they match*. Black T-shirt, black cotton pants or ankle-long black gauze skirt, multiflowered blouse as *jacket*. Belt in gold; add flat gold sandals. Or belt in red; add red sandals.

Blouse as a Jacket to Pull Together a Skirt and Sweater

• Beige turtleneck sweater, brown corduroy skirt, brown silk blouse as *jacket*. Belt in tone of brown leather. Add

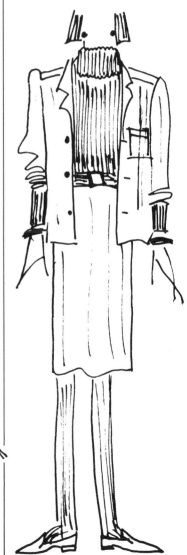

BLOUSE

brown ribbed opaque tights (the color of skirt) and matching brown flat shoes. A super-comfortable go-to-work look!

For Country

• Take three tones of *nut* colors: walnut corduroy jeans, vicuña-toned sweater, peanut silk blouse as *jacket*. Add short flat country boots. For dash, add a thin wool plaid shawl in shades of cream, beige to brown. Some of the prettiest

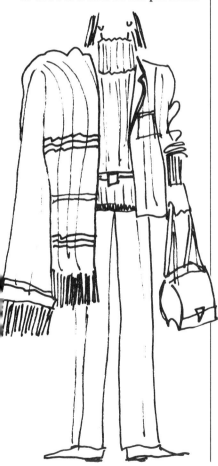

"shawls" are blankets meant for car blankets or day bed covers! Look for them in blanket and bed sitting room departments.

Evening

• Pale gray silk blouse as jacket plus gray flannel trousers over bare or strapless sweater-like tube top in cream wool knit. (Or a bare camisole top of dark cream silk jersey, or pale rose satin cut like lingerie. Note: Sometimes one can even find these "evening treasures" in lingerie departments!) Belt in metallic kid. Wear matching metallic sandals. Or do entire turnout in black: *Black* wool gabardine or velvet trousers, *black* silk blouse jacket over *scarlet* sweater-camisole or dark **violet** bare satin camisole. Belt with black satin ribbon bowed at the waist. Wear black satin sandals or pumps. Be sure if you wear pumps to add **sheer black stockings** to keep everything toned! If sandals, make sure you have well-pedicured toes—painted a shade of scarlet!

• Trick: Tie a blouse closed at the collar with a ribbon or cord of silk. Wear it open from the neck as a *jacket* over a pretty bare camisole for evening, a sweater and skirt, or a T-shirt and trousers for day!

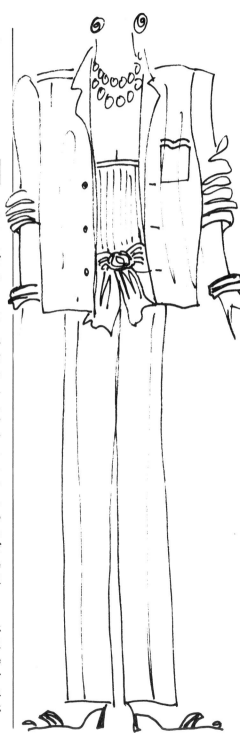

BASIC EVENING—WARDROBE

Fabrics

- Thin Silk/Crepe de Chine is ideal

- Silky Jersey (Remember, it is clingy—harder to wear)

- Satin Charmeuse (thin silk satin)

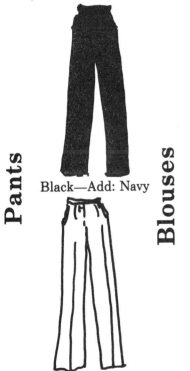

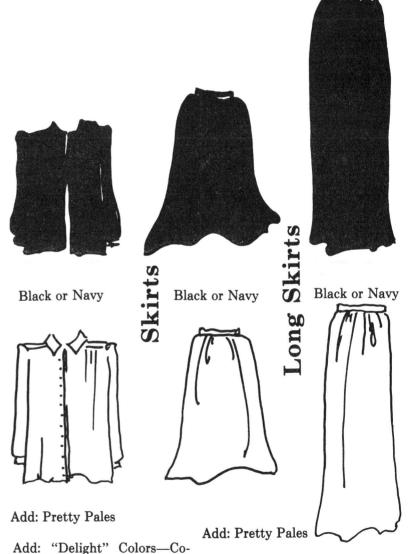

Pants

Black—Add: Navy

- Pretty Pale: Cream, Beige, Taupe, Pale Peach, Pale Gray, etc.

- Jewel Colors: Claret, Ruby, Dark Emerald

Blouses

Black or Navy

Add: Pretty Pales

Add: "Delight" Colors—Cobalt Blue, Crimson, Pale Pink, Scarlet

Skirts

Black or Navy

Add: Pretty Pales

Long Skirts

Black or Navy

- Jewel Colors: Claret, Ruby, Dark Emerald

Camisoles

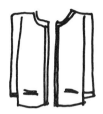

Black or Navy

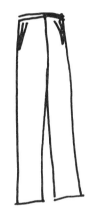

Add: Pretty Pales

• Jewel Colors
Add: "Delight" Colors—Cobalt Blue, Crimson, Pale Pink, Cream, Scarlet

Dinner Suits

Fabric: Satin, Velvet, Thin Wool, Crepe (less evening, but possible) or Silk Crepe

Pants

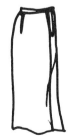

Black or Navy

Skirt

Black or Navy

Jackets

• Black

• Navy
Jacket Note: Stick to cardigan shape for evening. It moves as easily as a sweater does for day. A cardigan is a timeless classic!

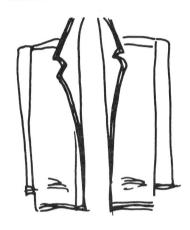

Extra Evening Jacket

• Scarlet

• Emerald

• Magenta
Pretty "Jewel" Color is key. Wear over anything as one would a jewel—to add "delight"!

BASIC EVENING WARDROBE

Evening Dress

• One "Big" Evening Dress
For the unexpected important night! Keep it soft, easy, *pretty* and dark-toned . . . this way it can stay in your life for seasons.
Black Georgette
Navy Thin Silk Satin
Dark Wine Silk Jersey

• One Evening Coat
⅞ is best—you can wear it over short dresses, long dresses, and trousers! Depending on where you live, look for soft quilting or a soft fur (preferably removable) as lining . . . This way your coat works winter as well as spring and fall.
Black Velvet
Black Satin
Fur
Black Cashmere wool with a ruby-quilted satin lining!

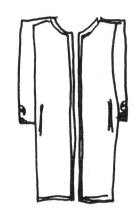

Shawl (at least 54″ square)

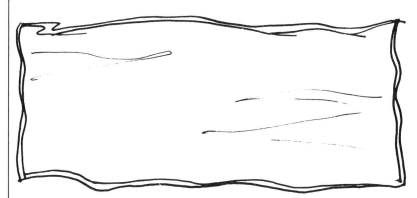

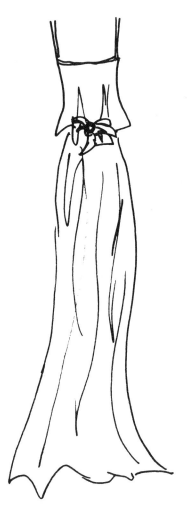

• Black Cashmere

• Dark Jewel-toned Paisley Wool

• Claret Cashmere/Silk

• Dark Crimson *Silk* (or any wonderful jewel color!) Fling a shawl over your shoulder for warmer nights, or wear it to add dash to your evening coat. Wear *indoors*, as an accessory.

It is the perfect and alluring lift to your black silk camisole-and-trouser evening pajama look! Remember: it must be big enough to really "wrap" into and thin and soft enough to use alone in warmer weather as well as to wrap *over* coat for an additional layer of warmth on a blizzardy evening!

More on Shawls: See Basic Scarf Wardrobe Section

• **For a successful evening wardrobe,** choose pieces in late-day fabrics: silk, crepe de chine, silk jersey, silk crepe, velvet, satin. The reason: *you have already built a skeleton wardrobe with wool, gabardine and other day fabrics.* These new pieces in evening fabrics will also be used to turn **day looks into evening** looks! For example, nothing looks prettier than a black cashmere sweater (day) over a silk skirt (evening). Waist-tie it with a black satin ribbon and you have a great look for drinks or dinner in a restaurant!

• As with **Basic Day Wardrobe,** always try to *match* as many pieces as possible. Trousers, skirt, blouse, bare top, long skirt, all in the same fabric and color, will give you instantly:

• Trouser + Blouse = Evening Pajama

• Trouser + Bare Top = more festive, *sexy* Evening Pajama

• Skirt + Blouse = Dinner Dress

• Skirt + Bare Top = Dance Dress

• Long Skirt + Bare Top = Big Evening Look—Black-Tie

• Long Skirt + Blouse = Dinner Dress for a Black-Tie, Formal, Conservative Evening.

• *Start with black* (or navy *if you feel best in navy).* Black or navy can go anywhere! Black or navy is timeless *and* seasonless. You add the color and glitter with accessories. *Then begin collecting.* Add pieces of a pretty, skin-flattering **pale color** (pale peach, silver gray, creamy beige, soft smoky pale taupe). *Make sure you buy all the pieces available in your pale tone as you did with your black or navy.* Or if you prefer, instead of a pale color add pieces in a jewel color: darkly beautiful gem tones, ruby, sapphire blue, dark emerald.

KEY: These must be skin-flattering tones! Remember, **evening is a personal time**—you must *Feel* wonderful to *Look* wonderful! *Whatever you buy for evening has to meet this test:* You must feel *beautiful* in it. Otherwise it is not worth any price. You will never feel comfortable or attractive; you will never therefore look your best. **Tip:** Remember all evening colors will be seen in *evening* (electric, candle, etc.) *light.* Do not be fooled by a pretty tone in daylight. Colors can wash out or change in night light. If you are not sure, ask the store sales person to find you a non-day-lit spot in which to check colors **before** you buy.

• Do the same for the dinner suit as you did for the silk pieces: in an *evening fabric match* jacket, pants, and skirt if you can. So you have:

• **An "extra" jacket** for evening to turn a wool trouser and sweater into an evening look or to put over a silk dress as an evening cover.

• **A good evening skirt-suit** look for theatre, restaurants, art exhibit openings, and business dinners.

• **An evening trouser-suit** . . . a great way to look at a restaurant, at the theater, or for drinks at someone's home. Art gallery openings: Again *black is best.* A black velvet turnout can serve you for years!

Evening Tricks: Slide one of the bare camisole tops of silk (dark or pale) under your velvet jacket and skirt or trousers—a fabulous look and especially pretty when you slip the jacket off at dinner!

Wear the "dinner suit jacket" over silk pajamas or silk blouse, (or camisole) and skirt. Wear one of your pretty day blouses or a bare sweater with dinner trouser suit look.

BASIC EVENING WARDROBE

- *The "Extra Evening Jacket"*: This piece is meant to be a delight in your evening wardrobe, a jewel. *It should be* beautiful! Make sure, to insure longlife and mobility, that it is an easy *classic shape*. You will want to slide it over dresses—long and short—evening pajamas, *bare* dresses, even a sweater and gray flannel trousers in the evening. *Think cardigan!* A cardigan works over anything and is a good shape for most bodies. Make sure that it is a *beautiful* color. Jewel and pale colors become "neutrals" at night! You can wear red, emerald, as well as cream or pale peach over black, navy, brown, dark gray as you would a fabulous bracelet! **Key:** *A jacket such as this becomes an accessory*; you use it to enliven, add dash and color, make a "Look" look and feel festive and extra attractive!

General Rules Basic Evening Wardrobe

- Always buy the best fabric and workmanship possible (the usual rule!). Not only will the parts look and perform better, you will *feel* better, more "expensive" in them, which is the key since evening is an especially beautiful time! Also the pieces will *work* for you longer. They will last psychologically as well as physically.

- After the **basic foundation** is set, begin collecting pieces which can **interplay** with them: bare silky tops in wonderful "color" colors, more blouses in "color" colors . . . maybe add one great pair of trousers in dark wine velvet or satin, or white silk if you live in a "summer place," or dark violet silk (to wear with a black sweater and your black velvet jacket, for instance). One begins to see the possibilities now—*it's called embellishing*. Result: You have begun an extremely versatile evening wardrobe which will work *any* season, anywhere, for a long long time.

- Note: This **Basic Evening Wardrobe** is designed to cover most situations in a life where evening dressing is as important, frequent, and varied as day. If you rarely dress in more than silk pants and a pretty shirt, you will know where to build and where not to bother.

  As with the Basic Day Wardrobe, it has also been worked out with a temperate climate in mind.

- *If you live in a warm place,* you may want to start building the silky section in a beautiful *pale* tone and then add a *second* pale. The **dinner suit** might be beige silk shantung, taupe crepe de chine, or cream silk crepe. The **extra jacket** could be silk in a wonderful skin-flattering color. The **long big-evening dress** could be dark rose or cream, pale smoke or beige, or peach-colored silk; **the shawl**, a huge 54″ square of red silk or a Gauguinesque flower print, or a giant square of smoky chiffon. You probably won't need the evening coat.

CAUTION: If you are heavy or have a figure problem, stick to dark tones—dark wine, perhaps, if you would rather not wear black! Remember, dark minimizes—light attracts! If you can't wear the pajama look of blouse tucked into trouser, look for a *silky tunic* that falls loose and straight to mid-thigh to wear over matching trousers. Try to find a *narrow*

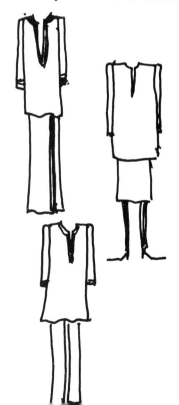

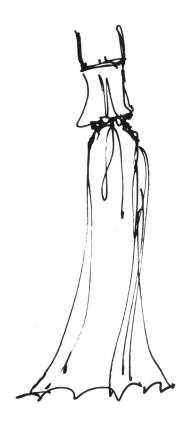

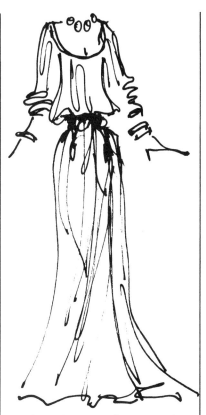

matching short skirt and also one to-the-floor over which the tunic will slide attractively!

• *If you live in the country,* you might substitute thin *knitted cashmere or wool jersey* for the silk section.

• You may not need a velvet dinner suit, but a **dark-toned wool jersey** one could be handy to wear with silky or bare sweaterlike tops!

• You may want to collect **velvet and satin trousers,** however, to wear with pretty blouses and sweaters—or a big

tunic pajama and pants of a lovely color of **knitted angora and wool** or cashmere.

• **The shawl** could be a huge, plaid, thin wool blanket or one of alpaca and wool or the knitted cashmere one from day. You would probably eliminate the bare *long dress* but have a long thin wool or silk jersey one with sleeves instead . . . or a bare floor-length knitted tube of a dress (a "sweater to the floor") over which to wear a cardigan sweater when it gets cool. *The Extra Evening Jacket* might be of scarlet *knitted* cashmere!

• *Know your evening needs.* Make sure you have something on hand to meet each major need, something in which you *look and feel* wonderful!

• **Make sure you have all the perfect evening accessories** to *complete every look*: bag, shoe/stocking, belt, *make-up*! *Rehearse* this part. One hour before you go out is not the time to discover you don't have a belt to tie up your Georgette dress or that the only sandals you own are black and your dress is pale cream. **TIP:** Try to keep all the evening accessories—bag, belt, shoe, etc.—per outfit either with the outfit or together in a separate bag marked "Navy Georgette Dress" or "Black Velvet Bag, Black Satin Shoe, Satin Belt."

• When you buy a *bare* top, be sure you own the *bra* to wear with it. If you don't own one, buy it at the same time you buy the top. You can try them on together for fit. This saves the last-minute surprise of not having the right bra, therefore not being able to wear the "divine top"!

REHEARSE. *Try* out the complete look—lingerie and all— when you have time (a Saturday afternoon). *Try out any new makeup then!* Try on all new purchases to make sure there are no hem adjustments needed and that everything hangs evenly. **Tip:** *Do this also* with anything you've owned for a while and haven't worn. The slim-legged silk trousers have a way of being less slim than you imagined if you haven't tested them for a season or so.

Trick: Keep your evening bag filled with evening essentials: a tiny powder compact, lipstick or gloss (enough for a touch-up), haircomb, one $5 bill (emergency taxi), some dimes (for pay phones!), a few quarters (for ladies' room tips), *an extra set of house and car keys!* This saves that last-minute fumble for those essentials *and* the awful surprise of walking out the door and forgetting the house keys!

• *Instant Evening* for when you arrive home from the office ten minutes before your escort or your guests are due! You're already in gray flannels and a gray sweater. Off with your heeled moccasins, on with gold sandals. Add a soft crushed-gold belt, some attractive gold bracelets and earrings. Slide a **colored** evening cover over all: a magenta shawl, a pale peach silk blouse worn as a jacket, or a rust velvet jacket. **Where to Spend Time:** A good ten minutes on a *makeup refresh.*

Makeup Reviver. If you

can't do a redo, begin with a fine spray of mineral water to revive your face. It doesn't remove makeup *if* you pat dry *gently!* This will make you *feel* prettier. Then rub a pad of cotton dipped in cologne around your hairline, back of neck, over ears, even along the part in your hair . . . a freshening relaxer!

Tip: If you're tired, for the first drink of the evening try a tomato juice instead of alcohol. It will give you a hit of good energy (potassium) instead of the head swimmer of alcohol!

• **Reviver Trick:** When you don't have time to shower before going out at night (face it, it *does* happen occasionally!) a dusting of nicely scented talcum will give you a lift.

Wardrobe Tip: To avoid last-minute panic, always have a supply of sheer black and sheer leg-color *sandalfoot* stockings on hand to avoid finding runs in every pair you put on when you are in a rush!

Tip: If you are wearing sandals at night, *always remember to check toes.* Make sure your nail polish is not chipped. Nothing looks worse than ungroomed toes peaking out from evening sandals when you are all done up! Make sure you have your nail polish color on

hand for a quick touch-up. The time to do it is **before makeup** so it has time to dry!

• *The key to evening dressing—Perfect finish!* This means:

Hair
Makeup
Hands
Feet

• *Hair must look wonderful!* If it doesn't learn how to "fake it." Learn the tricks! Slick it back. Pin a fresh flower in it. Wear important earrings (if you can carry the look): To embellish, do an extra-super makeup! For more hair ideas see Hair Section. For scarf tricks see Scarf Section.

• *Makeup at night is major,* not only to complete your look but because **night lighting** is hard on skin, draining to color! You must know how to counteract it in order not only to look your best but to look Extra-Wonderful.

• **Remember:** Jewelry at night and bare glittery shoes attract the eye to your face, your hands, your feet. **Beautifully groomed hands and feet are essential!** Lacquered toenails! Even if your hands look better with clear polish and white-stick under nails, toenails should be beautifully colored if they show.

Formulas: Twenty-Nine Ways to Use Basic Evening Wardrobe

You'll likely discover more!

Note: For clarity we will do the workout with one basic color family, black, and one second color family, pale peach.

Note: Refer to Belts, Shoes, Basic Jewelry Wardrobe, Basic Handbag Wardrobe and Basic Scarf Wardrobe sections for more accessory variations.

1. Black satin trousers + black silk blouse = *evening pajama*.

Add: Gold belt, gold sandals, gold-and-emerald-colored jewels.

2. Black silk skirt + black silk blouse = *dinner dress*.

Add: Black satin sandals, gold-and-black satin belt, gold and garnet jewels!

3. Black silk skirt + bare camisole = *dance dress*.

Add: Gold sandals, gold belt, pretty jewels, plus a 54″ square of black-and-red silk chiffon as a shawl. Wonderful black-tie dinner-restaurant look.

4. Black bare camisole + long skirt = *evening dress*.

Add: Gold sandals, gold-and-black satin belt, gold and rhinestone jewels. Major black-tie evening look.

5. Black silk blouse + long black silk skirt = *covered black-tie dinner dress*.

Add: Black-satin-and-gold belt, black satin sandals (or dark red satin sandals and belt). Ideal look for convention/business dinners, black-tie dinner at someone's home, etc. Add a dark red cashmere or silk blanket-shawl as an evening cover.

6. Black silk bare camisole + black silk trousers = *bare evening pajama*.

Add pale peach silk blouse as jacket, dark scarlet silk kimono-jacket, or a 54″ square of red-and-black-printed silk! With black-and-gold belt, black satin or gold kid sandals, you have a great look for a museum opening, dinner party, cocktails, etc.

7. Pale peach blouse + black silk pants = *evening pajama look*.

Add a belt of black satin ribbon tied in a bow at center front waist. Tuck a fresh pale pink camellia into bow. Open blouse as much as you dare (*or* wear the black silk camisole *or* matching peach silk camisole underneath and open blouse to waist). Add black satin sandals, gold and rock crystal beads, gold earrings!

8. Pale peach silk camisole + pale peach silk long skirt = *black-tie evening, summer, winter, anywhere*.

If you want to look fragile and extra-pretty, add gold sandals, gold belt, and pale rose quartz jewelry. Keep everything pale!

9. Pale peach blouse + pale peach short skirt = *dinner dress*.

Lovely for afternoon weddings, convention/business dinners where you want to look attractive and keep a conservative edge. Add gold. You have a seasonless look—summer, winter, anywhere!

10. Black velvet jacket + peach silk camisole = black velvet skirt = *dinner suit*.

Add: Black satin pumps, tiny black satin bag, gold jewels. Terrific look for theater or cocktails in any big city in the world!

11. Black velvet jacket and black velvet trousers + ivory cashmere crewneck sweater or cream silk blouse (from day wardrobe). Add black satin sandals, black satin ribbon bowed at waist, gold bangles, earrings. Great easy-evening dinner suit look, for restaurants, theater, etc.

12. Black velvet jacket + black velvet skirt + black silk camisole = *dinner suit*. Add gold jewels, gold belt, black satin sandals. For a "touch," pin a small white gardenia to your lapel. Looks especially beauti-

ful when you remove your jacket at the table; the bare silk camisole is so attractive!

13. Black velvet jacket + cream cashmere sweater + gray flannel pants = *easy evening*. Add gold belt, sandals.

14. Black velvet jacket + black silk bare camisole + brown tweed trousers + gold belt + brown kid sandals = another *sexy* easy evening! For Dash, carry a **Dark Red Kid Evening Bag**!

15. Black velvet jacket over black silk blouse + black silk skirt = *the perfect evening cover*.

16. Black velvet jacket over peach silk camisole and peach silk trousers = another great-looking *evening cover*.

17. Black velvet jacket over black cashmere crewneck sweater + brown tweed trousers = *great easy evening*! Add brown belt, brown kid sandals, gold jewelry.

18. Black crewneck cashmere sweater + black velvet trousers + gold belt + gold sandals = *divine easy evening look*. Add a gardenia tucked into belt, gold jewelry, big black cashmere shawl.

19. Black cashmere crewneck sweater + black velvet skirt. Add black satin pumps, black satin-and-gold belt. Substitute lots of gold jewelry for flower. Throw a dark red shawl over

your shoulder as an evening cover. Great theater, restaurant, cocktail party look.

20. Black cashmere crew sweater + its cardigan + black silk skirt = *easy extra-pretty restaurant dinner look*. Add black satin ribbon-bowed waist (tuck a camellia in bow if you like!), black satin sandals, gold jewels.
The cardigan is the evening cover!

21. Magenta satin "extra evening jacket" + black silk camisole + black silk trousers = *terrific evening pajama cover*.

22. Magenta satin jacket + black velvet skirt + black silk bare camisole (black satin ribbon bowed at waist) + black satin shoes = *super dinner look*. Can go to a restaurant dinner, theater opening, etc.

23. Magenta satin jacket + gray cashmere sweater + gray flannel trousers = smashing easy evening look!
Add gold belt, sandals, gold jewelry.

24. Magenta satin jacket + peach silk bare camisole + peach silk long skirt = *ideal evening cover*.

25. Magenta satin jacket + cream silk shirt + black gabardine trousers = *smashing easy evening*.
Add black satin sandals, black satin ribbon bowed at waist + gold jewelry. Or, try a gold

chain with a jeweled buckle.

26. Magenta satin jacket + cream silk blouse + *black velvet trouser or skirt = great dinner suit look*.
Add black satin sandals and ribbon bowed at waist.

27. Magenta satin jacket over black georgette big evening dress = *beautiful evening cover*.

28. Black velvet 7/8 cardigan "evening coat" over all evening looks listed above. Especially chic: black velvet coat + black cashmere sweater + brown tweed trousers. Add: Black satin sandals, black satin ribbon bowed at waist, gold jewels. In Paris, London, New York, Chicago, San Francisco, the perfect way to go to dinner in a restaurant, drinks after work, theater, movies/late supper date, etc.!

29. Black velvet 7/8 coat + black velvet skirt + bare black silk camisole + black satin sandals + ribbon bow waist + gold = *museum opening, concert, restaurant dinner party!*

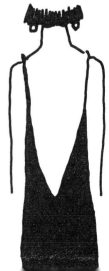

EVENING MAKEUP

The trick: Intensify!

Before doing the makeup change:

1. SPEND TWO MINUTES RELAXING. Lie down with feet higher than head. Do deep breathing to get oxygen in, toxins out! (See detensing exercise section.)

2. *Intensify eye color.* With a brush dipped in a smoky tone, run color (against skin grain) outside edge lower lid, toward nose, then outside edge upper lid toward nose, then back along upper lid and up and around to eyelid crease. Then along eyelid crease toward nose. (Note: You are making a circular movement with brush on upper lid.)

3. *Intensify Mascara.* Gently recurl lashes. Reapply mascara. Brush out each layer. Apply, brush out, apply, etc. Separate lashes at last application.

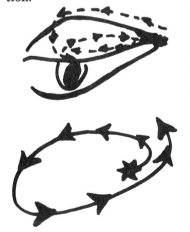

4. *Intensify Cheeks.* Add more cheek color with a brush and *powder blush* this time. Concentrate color on cheekbone towards temples. *Powder is better now as you are contouring and intensifying over your day color.* It doesn't remove foundation, etc! Don't forget a dash of color on earlobes!

5. *Highlight.* With a clean brush, dust some gold powder at sides of forehead near hairline, just under chin, along outside of cheekbones near hairline. Apply just a touch in the *center* of *each upper eye* lid to "hold it all together"! Then, gently dust finishing powder just a touch on lids to diffuse the added eye color.

6. *Intensify Mouth. Reline your mouth.* Apply a more intense color at inside center of lips only. Use a shade lighter toward the edges. Blend. Apply gloss only to *center of mouth*! This makes for a rounder, more sensuous and *less shiny mouth. Remember: night lighting makes overly glossy lips look plastic*! Therefore, apply gloss only at the center of lips!

Makeup Tips

1. *At Night*: Hair, makeup, hands, feet can make or break—a "look"! This is the time to be "perfect"!

2. Lighting — Color Tips:
• *Florescent light* (in offices, etc.) drains color—emphasizes blues. If you spend a lot of time in florescent lights, stay away from colors with blue tones such as purples or blues-reds, berry colors, violets. Keep tones in the family of warm golden tawny colors (apricot, peach, etc.). Remember to keep foundation skin tones warm also . . . not overly whitened.

• *Incandescent* (at night) emphasize yellows. Do the opposite of day: Keep makeup colors *away* from yellowy bronzes and tawny tones. Go for roses and bordeauxs, berries violets. Keep skin tone paler (ivoried)—eyes stronger. Balance eye-color strength with more cheek and mouth color (or you will risk looking cadaverous!).

3. Night Makeup Tip: In night light, too much shine on skin looks hot and sweaty. *Keep makeup matte.* Keep powdering *lightly* with a brush and loose translucent powder through an evening.

4. Evening Trick: A tiny *dab* of your *lip* color at the *center* of upper eyelids—to "centralize and balance" everything! Try it!

5. TRICK: For fuller, natural-looking lips, put a dab of cream blusher or dark-toned lip color at the *inside* center of

upper and lower lips. Then gloss lips all over to blend. The effect—like "sucking on a strawberry popsicle"—is a beautifully rounded, sensual and natural mouth.

6. TAKE A LAST LOOK: Before leaving home, check your face in a magnifying mirror. Look for uneven lines, smudges . . . too much or too little or imbalanced color!

7. TIP: Powder for Day: For a natural, unpowdery look, try applying powder with a *damp* silk sponge. Shake some loose powder onto a small plate. Dip in sponge. (This keeps powderbox from getting caky.) Dab—press, release, press, release action on face.

8. Trick—Day Mouth: For a natural, unlipstick-looking mouth, mix lip color first with clear gloss and then apply to lips with a brush.

9. Cover Trick: Try a paler *foundation* tone rather than cover stick to lighten dark areas. Foundation texture is lighter, less masklike, especially good if skin texture isn't smooth. (for instance crepey under eye areas!). Apply lightly. Dab and pat!

10. Trick for eye makeup: A light brush of translucent powder over lids pales and diffuses eye makeup delicately!

11. *At-Home Night Lighting Trick*: Put pink bulbs in your lamps. Makes light rosy . . . infinitely more flattering!

12. Remember—Jewelry Attracts the Eye: Make sure that your hands are perfectly groomed if you are wearing bracelets and rings. Make sure that your makeup is beautifully finished—mouth and eyes and cheeks "balanced" with color!—if you wear earrings, necklaces! This is as important as clean hair, clean skin, face, and hands!

Warm Weather Tips: Instead of foundation wear a sunscreen. Then mix a little *moisturizer* with a cream blush (makes it thinner, more transparent). Dab blush on sides of forehead, cheeks, chin, under jawbone for a healthy glow. Great trick for winter-pale skin!

More Evening Touches

1. For Effect: A touch of highlighter—the palest tone of your eyeshadow (or *if* you have an expert hand try a silvered or gold highlighter!) Dot a speck at the corners of eyes (the outside corners if your eyes are close-set—at the inside corners if they are far-set!) . . . Dot a speck at the corners of your mouth! It lifts the edges. A dab along top of cheekbones (near temples!) . . . at hairline, at the sides of forehead. A touch at base of neck where collarbones meet . . . on tops of shoulderbones (for bare dressing!). A dab on backs of hands (makes your dinner table ges-

tures look wonderful)! These points will catch light, and sparkle!

2. Run blush onto earlobes . . . or a dab of lipgloss on lobes for shine—but gloss only if your are wearing your hair back! Makes earrings look even more effective!

3. Try a finishing powder with sheer glimmer added (gold or silver-flecked)! A thin, delicate woosh with a brush over face—ear lobes, sides of neck, chest, over shoulder bones for gleam! *Note: Keep gleam off nose*—it is the first place to have its own! "Set" powder by *gently* patting with finger tips. Moisture of fingers helps the setting.

4. The best summer foundation: water-based rather than oil-based. It allows skin to breathe; it's thinner, less clogging to pores. Summer heat enlarges pores!

- **Tip:** "Dilute" foundation with moisturizer for a *thinnest* veil of covering!
- **Tip:** If you use pencils for eyes, lips etc., keep them in the *refrigerator before sharpening.*
- Keep cologne, a spray bottle of mineral water (your wake-up splasher) in *refrigerator.*
- Use powder colors rather than creams! They won't melt.
- Have your lashes dyed to eliminate mascara smudging problems.

SCENT

The Way to Apply:

Your personal touch... your image and reflection. The most effective places to use fragrance are at pulse points: wrists, throat, bosom, inner arms, back of knees, neck, etc., but *not* behind ears!

TIP: Always apply your fragrance *before* putting on jewelry! Oils can damage stones, pearls, etc. Never spray on furs! It dries skins!

Fragrance Routine: for Maximum Effect

• Begin with the bath-oil version in your morning tub.

• Then spray on cologne *after* bath while your body is still warm and damp. Afterward, towel dry.

• About a half hour before going out, apply the perfume version to your pulse points. This gives the scent time to grow and to settle!

Important: Reapply perfume or cologne often during the day. At least every three to four hours, the fragrance wanes and effects ebb! General rule: Keep sultry, musky, heavy scents for night. Use fresh, clean, light ones for day. *Do not* apply a fresh application of fragrance before going into a restaurant or into dinner. It can be a bit much with food smells.

Tricks with Scent

• Spray cologne on feet (through stockings) often during day and evening. It diffuses around in clouds as you walk and is also a great "reviver."

• **At home,** fill a basin with *hot* water. Add a good amount of your scent in its bath oil form. Let it stand for hours! It makes your atmosphere smell delicious! (and personal!)

• Trick: A perfume-scented handkerchief or sachet is a lovely trick in your handbag. When you open your bag to powder your nose, pay the taxi, etc., clouds of your scent filter out. Great for crowded trains!

• Spray your fragrance on the hems of your clothes. As you walk, more clouds come up!

• Lightly spray on hair, especially in summer! Try spraying some on *damp* hair—the fragrance penetrates better as hair dries.

For More "Atmosphere"

• Put sachets or cotton balls saturated with your favorite perfume oil in your suitcases while in storage. When you pack for a trip, your clothes will pick up the fragrance!

• Tuck oil or perfume-soaked cotton balls behind chair and couch cushions. When you sit down, clouds of scent are released.

• Put sachets, etc., in drawers, and tuck into corners of closets. When you open and close them, fragrance wafts out.

• Spray radiators, curtains—even rugs—with your favorite scent. Heat and movement through a room release the scent!

• Spray air conditioners, or for maximum effect, saturate a tissue and tape onto air-conditioning grate. Slit tissue a few times with a knife so that air can pass through! When air conditioner is on it propels the scent through your rooms.

• Tricks for the loveliest sleep:

• A *light* spray of cologne on your body before putting on your nightgown. Tuck sachets or scent-laden cotton balls way down between sheets and bed. When you open the bed to get in, there is a delicious cloud!

• Spray the inside of your terry bathrobe. When you slip into it damp from your bath—more loveliness! This is great trick for wearing fragrance in the sun, you don't risk pigment spots if you: spray the inside of your beach cover-up.

• Put a few drops of perfume oil on a small asbestos ring.

SCENT

You can buy these in candle shops or soap and fragrance departments. Place on light bulbs. The heat of the bulbs releases fragrance into the atmosphere. Lovely!

• Tuck sachets, perfume-scented cotton balls, or scented soap at bottom of laundry bag or baskets.

• Cut up desk blotters and saturate with your fragrance. Tuck them everywhere you want a surprise of fragrance—in drawers, behind cushions, behind books. Use the strips as bookmarks!

• Keep a basket of scented soap open in your bathroom. Moisture and the heat of water will release scent!

TRAVEL TIP: Bring along scented soap, sachets, and asbestos rings to scent and put on light bulbs. Remember a spray of cologne on hotel curtains, bathroom curtains, in closets, drawers, etc., to make it *"your* room!"

• Spray ironing board with your cologne before ironing lingerie, blouses, handkerchiefs, etc.—This way, you "press in" your fragrance!

Recipe for Instant, Delicious Atmosphere

Fill a saucepan of water. Add a handful of dried whole cloves and one cinnamon stick. Bring to a boil on stove. Then allow it to simmer. The longer you simmer, the more delicious the smell throughout your house! Caution: Check often for water evaporation and add water if needed!

REVIVERS AND RELAXERS

Fact: There is no way that you can ignore any part of your body. A pretty makeup will not do much for you if you are tight, tense or fatigued. Fact: *Your entire body operates as a single mechanism*: when it's healthy, in top form, and relaxed, every part of you reflects that state. Your hair, your skin, your nails, your voice, the way you *move, the way you interact with people* are all affected by your health and physical state. When you feel tense and tired you can never look and act peak-attractive.

The following are some tips on how to work a little instant magic and move into top form.

How to Get Out of Bed

• A Begin-the-Day-Tip: *Before you get out of bed, stretch like a cat!* Inhale deeply while on your back. Throw your pillow away so you lie flat. Stretch one leg down toward bottom of bed while the arm on the same side stretches towards top of bed. Hold for a count of five. Exhale. Repeat on other side. Do this a few times each side. *This is an easy and great body stretch*;

the deep breathing oxygenates your blood and tissues and gets your body going. It is the healthy way to get out of bed!

"Wake-up" Shower (good anytime—not only A.M.): Start with warm water. Slowly turn water down to nearly cold, then warm again, ending with nearly cold. *You're awake!*

Detensing Shower: While standing under a brisk jet of warm water, (1) hold stomach muscles in, (2) breathe deeply, and (3) lean over from waist, arms dangling loosely. Relax everywhere—arms, head, back, etc., except for stomach muscles. They must be held in—they support your body! Let the shower jet "beat" on the nape of your neck and down your spine . . . across your shoulders . . . on all the key tension spots! It feels *wonderful*!

Two-Minute Mid-Morning Reviver: *No coffee! Yes, exercise!* Stand with feet apart. Stomach muscles in. Inhale deeply. Put hands on shoulders, elbows out, at a 90-degree angle to body. Swing right arm in a windmill motion in a circle *downward* while you turn your torso to the right and stretch your left arm as far back as possible. Exhale. *Do not move legs and hips*; only the torso and arms turn and swing. Return to starting position facing front, hands on shoulders. Inhale. Repeat turning left, right arm back as far as possible. Exhale. Keep doing this movement, right, left, right, left (without pausing in between!), *and*, **most important, while** *breathing deeply* **and** *rhythmically*! Inhale at start, front. Exhale to right. Inhale front. Exhale left. Do this for 1–2 minutes. You are oxygenating your blood, which means better circulation, which means instant energy!

Bath Revivers

Bath Energizer

For a lift, take a cool bath (65°–75°F) for 10 minutes—no longer! The cool water helps stimulate circulation. Note on baths: *Hot* water is definitely not good for you! It dries and ages the skin, injures delicate capillaries and veins. It is debilitating and weakening!

Bath Relaxer
A warm bath (85°–95°F) is a relaxer! Trick: Make an "atmosphere" before getting in the bath. Keep lights low or try a bath-by-candlelight! Put your favorite bubble bath in the tub. Light a scented candle. Put on soft music. Then rest in the water for 15 minutes. **Tip:** If your skin is the least bit dry, *always add bath oil to the water or rub your body down gently with a body moisturizer or oil before* getting into the tub!

Bath Recipes

Morning Bath:
Soak 7 minutes in a seaweed or algae bath. Just before getting out, run *cool* (not cold!) water into tub. Good for circulation! **Makeup trick:** Apply your foundation and eyeshadow *before* getting into your bath. The moisture helps "set" these "bases" and keeps makeup looking fresher longer! **Bath for winter-dry skin:** Add 3 lbs. of oatmeal (tied in a muslin bag) to your bath! Swish it around and tie it onto the faucet. Soak for 15 min-

utes. Soothing! **For blood circulation:** Gently rub your body down with a damp loofa sponge before getting into the tub. Apply a light layer of body moisturizer, then soak in the oatmeal bath!

Night Baths:

Cleanse face and apply a mask. Take a sulfur bath to ease muscle tension. Soak 10 minutes. To revive a little after this relaxing bath, add cool water to tub before you get out.

Sleep-Inducing Bath: Put on soft music. Add your favorite scented bubble bath. Moisturize body well before getting into water. *Drink a glass of warm milk* while soaking. Soak 10 minutes—no longer! Dry off and go right to bed.

• *Instant Reviver Fragrance!* **Rub back of neck and hairline with cologne— fresh from the refrigerator is best!** Keep a bottle *there for last-minute* lifts, especially in summer. Spray some on back of knees inside of arms, at elbows . . . *feet!* Spray a little "veil" in hair— wonderful lift!

• **Skin Reviver:** Ice cubes. If skin is sensitive or dry, wrap cubes in thin cotton or a tissue! Rub a few lightly over your face, neck, back of neck. Don't forget wrists. This helps reduce puffiness around eyes, tightens facial pores . . . And it's a great morning awakener! If tiny wrinkles are a problem—especially around eyes—apply a light touch of oil first. Castor oil is wonderfully mild for this.

• **For Eyes:** A splash of cold water! A *fine spray* from a refrigerated spray bottle (or can) of mineral water. A great midday tip—it doesn't remove makeup and makes you feel instantly energized!

Trick—Hair Reviver: Set your hair *before* getting into your tub or shower. The steam helps make it curl more quickly.

• **FACE DETENSER:** Great after a long jaw-clenching day! Lie down on your back, feet up, mind "cooled down." Some Vivaldi on the stereo will help! Place a cork (the wine bottle kind) between your teeth. Do *not* bite down! Just hold the cork between your teeth *gently* while you close your eyes for *10 minutes* and *breathe rhythmically.* Amazing results! Your face will look weekend-fresh and your whole body will have relaxed. Do this, if you have

time, *before* putting on evening makeup. Your face will be smoother and take makeup better. You will look even more sensational!

• **LIQUID REVIVERS:**
  • **Drink a glass of water.** Try it, it works!

  • **A cup of camomile tea.** Especially good after a tension-filled day! It's a relaxer.

  • *To restore potassium* especially after physical exertion and *especially* in heat: beef bouillon, orange juice, a banana! Often when you feel weak and "zapped" of energy it is because your potassium level has fallen. **Note:** Do not fall for the sugar "up." It is a false "up" and you will fall down quickly again. Also, who needs the calories!

• **Reviver:** Instant Beauty Trick: Think posture! Make it a habit. Back straight. Abdominal muscles in. Hips tucked under. Shoulders back and down. Arms free to swing. Head high, as if the top of your head was held to the ceiling by a string! *Whenever you remember, concentrate on this . . . as many times as possible in a day.* It is a tension-reliever too! You are immediately taking pressure off organs, your spine, etc. You

are rebalancing your body, which helps your blood to flow.

Midday Reviver: *A walk around the block!* • Do it *without* taking your handbag so your arms are free to swing.
• Walk *briskly*, arms swinging loosely from shoulders . . .
• Think about it! Your arms must be free to move in order to help release back and shoulder tension. • Stomach is held in, head is held high (to free any neck tension), back is aligned . . . in short, perfect marching posture. • Breathe deeply and rhythmically the whole time you are walking. It sounds simple but it's an incredibly effective reviver exercise!

• **Instant Stress Relief:** Yawn! The key is how you yawn: begin with tiny ones, mouth closed, then a big one with mouth open. Let your lungs fill with air, your ribs expand to their fullest, your diaphragm open like an umbrella. This deep oxygenation is amazingly reviving and relaxing. Repeat a few times.

• **Deep Air Inhaling,** Lung-Filling Sighs: Exhale through nose with mouth closed until you have no more air left in lungs. Do several times. These are great tricks to practice before giving a speech, chairing a meeting, or before any tension-building situation!

• **Detension Exercise:** 2 minutes. (1) Stand up, stomach in, back aligned. Arms should be very loose and relaxed. Close your eyes. Clench and unclench your hands. Breathe deeply for 30 seconds so that you become "quiet." (2) Put your hands, one over the other, on the back of your head, fingers facing downward so that they just touch the center point where skull and neck join—the little depression at the top of neck. (3) Bring your elbows forward so that they nearly touch in front of your forehead. (4) Keep your back and hips aligned and very straight, stomach tight. This is very important! (5) Gently (*very, very* gently!) pull your head downward, chin toward chest, while keeping your shoulders pressing downward. You will feel a pull along the spinal cord and across your shoulders. Be *gentle* but keep the tension of the "pull." Hold 1 minute. Then gradually and *slowly*—while holding head forward, chin on chest—roll your body forward from the waist a little bit at a time, gently, slowly! (Think of a cat!) *Do not force!* Keep breathing deeply, always holding stomach in, *always* pressing shoulders downward. *Do not turn your head.* You can pull

the muscles in your neck in this position. Release hands slowly by simply dropping your arms down. Do not lift your head yet. Keep hanging forward, head down, while you move your legs apart (about 1½ feet). With your head as a weight, continue bending over (from hips now) arms hanging down, stomach pulled in. Go only as far as you can without straining. Dangle there for 1 minute. Breathe! Relax in that position—try! Try swaying the body **just a little** from side to side from the base of the spine. Return to the dangle position. Then, inhale deeply and *slowly* uncurl (*very slowly* or you will become dizzy!) using your abdominal muscles to help lift your body! This is a great spine stretch as well as a body and mind relaxer.

• **Reviver Trick:** Exercise your voice! Stand tall with your chest and chin high, stomach in, hips tucked under. Take in a fast *deep* breath as if you were sipping through a straw. Hold the breath. As you exhale *slowly*, hiss your breath out through your teeth. Hiss to a slow count of 20 to 30. With practice, you should finally be able to exhale to a count of 60. Do *not push* breath out, let it flow out gently! *A constant long low exhalation decreases tension*, relaxes your body entirely. And notice how much

lower, sexier, and easier your voice sounds!

• **Total Body Detenser:** *How to Learn to Relax:* In a quiet place, lie down on your back and close your eyes. Extend your legs (relaxed), arms straight at sides, palms up (relaxed). Breathe. Listen to your breathing. Tense your right hand. Relax it. Let it feel limp, heavy, warm. Then move to your forearm, then your upper arm, then your shoulder. Breathe deeply, slowly, rhythmically. Think: "Tense, Relax." Do the same on your left side. Begin with your hand, then your arm, then shoulder. *Think*: "Relax, Heavy, Limp." Then do it with your foot, your leg, your hip, on one side and then the other side. Keep telling each part to relax, to feel *limp, heavy, warm.* Then move up to your abdomen, then your chest. Think: "Limp, Loose, Heavy, Warm." End with forehead. Breathe slowly, deeply. Think *cool, quiet.* With 15 minutes of practice daily, in 2 weeks' time you should be able to do this exercise to revive your body in 1½ minutes! **Note:** The secret to this exercise is the word *"Think."* You must learn to focus your mind on your breathing and the words *relax, heavy, warm.* Once you can do this and block out all other thoughts and outside sounds, you will be amazed at the speed and effectiveness of this exercise.

• **Total Body Detenser #2:** Sit comfortably in a straight-back chair in a quiet place. Pull the shades, turn down the lights. Inhale *deeply*. Hold breath 5 seconds. Count: "1 relax, 2 relax, 3 relax, 4 relax, 5 relax." Exhale *slowly*. Use your abdominal muscles! Think "relax." *Tell* your muscles to relax. Concentrate on breathing and on the word "relax." Try to block out everything but "breathe" and "relax." Repeat 4 or 5 times.

• **Quick Energizer #1:** Jog in place for 1–2 minutes lifting knees high. Important: The key to this is to breathe rhythmically. This exercise is especially effective if you are feeling low. Reoxygenating and increasing circulation helps rid the body of toxins, makes you literally **feel better!**

• **Quick Energizer #2:** Do 50–100 jumping jacks. Breathe rhythmically! Counting out loud helps breathing and stamina. **Caution:** Never jump on a hard floor in bare feet. The safest way to jump is with running shoes or on a *very padded* flat surface. Never jump in any day shoes.

Maintenance Exercises to Do Anywhere

• *To firm inner thighs, stom-ach, hips*: While seated at a desk or table, place legs straight out in front of you, toes touching under side of desk. Tighten stomach and buttocks muscles. Press feet upward as if to lift desk from floor. Hold position and tension of muscles for 6 seconds. Relax. Repeat 6 times.

• To Do: While under the dryer, while driving in a car, plane, bus, etc.: *To flatten stomach*: Hold stomach muscles taut to the count of 10. Release. Repeat 20 times. *To tighten and firm buttocks*: Squeeze buttocks muscles taut. Hold 10 seconds. Relax and repeat 20 times. *To firm upper arms and chest muscles*: Press forearms against chair arms. Hold to count of 10. Release. Repeat 20 times. *To strengthen ankles, reduce tension in legs, help circulation*—great for a long plane trip: Extend legs. Rotate feet clockwise 10 times, counterclockwise 10 times. Keep stomach and buttocks taut while doing for **extra benefits!** Do wherever you feel cramped.

• **Invisible exercises** to do while standing in line for bus, movies, etc.: *For derriere*: Stand straight, arms loose at sides. Tighten muscles of left buttock. Hold 10 seconds. Release. Tighten right buttock. Hold 10 seconds. Release. Tighten both. Hold 10 sec-onds. Release. Repeat 15–20 times. *For abdomen*: Hold stomach taut. Count 10. Release. Repeat 20–40 times.

Bath Exercises

To strengthen leg muscles and upper arms: Sit up straight in the tub. Press feet against end of tub. Brace arms on side of tub. Slowly raise and lower hips. Do 5–10 times. *To firm abdomen*: Brace your head on a "bath-pillow" at the back of tub. Hold onto the sides of the tub. Carefully raise legs. While holding abdomen muscles taut, bend one knee and straighten. Bend other knee, straighten. Do 5–6 times. *To firm thighs and especially inner thighs*: Have a small, soft rubber ball handy (tennis ball to softball size). While sitting straight, knees flexed, feet planted firmly, place ball between knees. Press knees together while holding abdomen muscles taut. Hold 10 seconds. Release. Press again. Hold 10 seconds. Do 10 times.

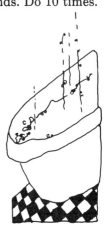

SPECIAL OCCASION DRESSING

The following are some of the situations in which one most frequently asks, "What do I wear?" The answers are guidelines suggestions which allow you "to take it from there" and do your own embellishing.

Some of the most difficult occasions to find "what to wear" are *Afternoon Events*—wedding, bar mitzvah, or graduation party, etc.

• A 7/8 long velvet coat or a velvet jacket over a *short crepe de chine dress* in a combination of pretty colors: a pale taupe silk dress/dark rust velvet coat or a pale peach silk dress/misty taupe-colored velvet jacket.

• For warmer weather, try crepe de chine cardigan jacket over a darker-toned silk jersey or silk crepe de chine dress: a dark apricot crepe de chine jacket over cocoa silk jersey, a cream crepe de chine jacket over taupe jersey, a rose crepe de chine jacket over navy silk.

• Another look: the **soft "suit."** A taupe jersey suit with makeup-pale rose silk camisole, a brown velvet suit with ivory silk bare blouse. Or

a bare dress and silky coat: a halter dress of cocoa silk and a loose kimono-coat of peach crepe de chine.

• A navy silk bare dress with narrow but softly gathered skirt, plus matching loose silky cardigan jacket or a cardigan jacket of black or dark wine velvet.

• *In summer or tropical places*: a pale flower-printed silk cardigan jacket over cream beige or ivory silk dress.

• A crepe de chine "suit": loose silky cardigan and matching softly gathered skirt with matching camisole top or one of another pale color, wheat-colored silk jacket and skirt, ivory camisole. Or: pale cocoa silk jacket and skirt and matching camisole. To make any of these look extra wonderful, add beautiful jewelry. For example, with the cocoa silk suit, wear pale pink quartz jewelry!

The point: A pretty, floaty covering over **a simple, easy, never fussy dress.** Let the color, tone and fabric do the work for you. Think

skin-flattering colors: apricot, powdery peach, rose, pale pinky-mauve. Balance pale, pretty tones with beiges, dark ivories, tones of gray—wonderful too with terracotta—rusty colors, navies.

SPECIAL OCCASION

Conference Lunch/Board Meeting/Banker-Lawyer Conference

• A navy jersey suit, colored (pale peach, pale blush) or white silk blouse! A brown jersey dress (see Dress Section) plus brown-toned tweed jacket, fur jacket, or brown-and-cream jersey cardigan.

• For warm places: a tan silk shantung or linen suit, with a white or pale peach silk blouse. A navy linen wrap dress, plus beige silk jacket. A peanut jersey sleeveless "T-shirt" top dress, plus cream linen jacket.

Black-Tie Convention Dinners, Embassy Receptions, Company Executive's Home Dinner

(Anywhere you want to be very attractive yet understatedly safe)

SPECIAL OCCASION DRESSING

• A short, *covered* dress in a *dark*-toned silky fabric, crepe de chine, thin soft jersey—"pretty" is key. A print, small, discreet on a dark background. See Dress Section for classic shapes. Or short, bare camisole dress in navy, wine or dark blueberry silk or a bare top and matching skirt (See Basic Wardrobe Evening.) of same dark-colored silky fabric with *matching silky cardigan* or kimono-shaped jacket as cover.

Black-Tie Opening Nights/Big City: Opera, Ballet, Theater

• Tunic jacket and matching trousers of pale taupe hammered satin, ivory satin, or thin gold lamé . . . black or dark-wine silk long-sleeved

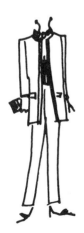

tunic over narrow black or dark-wine silk pants . . . cardigan jacket and skirt of velvet or black hammered satin over a dark rose or black bare top, a thin gold lamé jacket over bare satin dress.

Private Black-Tie Party—Holiday Time

• A sweater-shaped top and, long wrap skirt, or tunic pullover and pajama plus wonderful gold jewelry. *A fabulous color*: cobalt blue silk jersey, magenta or red silk, or white jersey belted in gold.

Convention Black-Tie Evening Or Black-Tie Executive Dinner Dance

• *Long, covered evening dress.* Think long sleeves, discreetly alluring, open neckline, long, easy skirt. Make the color and the fabric count: silver gray silk jersey, dark apricot silk, or banana-colored crepe. Save the glitter of gold lamé or dash of red satin for another occasion! Think simple and attractive: navy silk jersey long skirt and long-sleeved bateau-neck or nicely carved neck T-shirt top, black satin ribbon bowed at waist, a gardenia tucked into the knot—fabulous! Or: ankle-long, black, full bias chiffon skirt and matching long, full-sleeved blouse, with black satin ribbon belt, black satin sandals.

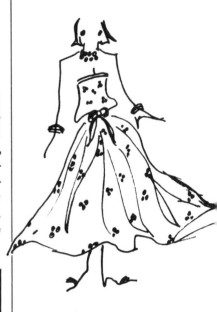

For Summer Dancing at a Country Club

• A bare-topped dress in a delicious color, or bare floor-length or ankle-length dress in tiny flower-printed silk or pale peach-and-cream stripe silk or a floaty tunic top and pajama of flowery chiffon. *Easy summer evening*: white cotton gauze strapless dress, full ankle-length skirt. Add gold belt, gold sandals. You have a very alluring look for dinner on someone's boat or island yacht club on a weekend.

BASIC JEWELRY —
WARDROBE

These are *guidelines* for building a jewelry collection that will work for you, as effortlessly, attractively, and magically as the basic wardrobe. Follow this guide and *add to your collection season after season.* You will continue to use and interchange all pieces and enrich looks with great success and pleasure.

DAY

Ears

Studs: Gold

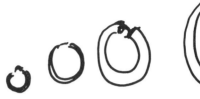

Hoops: Gold

Studs: Semiprecious stones and minerals, pearls   Add studs: Diamond set in gold

Wrists

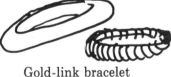

Gold-link bracelet

Gold bangles in several widths

Wood bangles and cuffs of inlayed wood, ivory, jade, etc.

Necks

Necklaces of semiprecious stones. Collarbone lengths and long ropes to hang in necklines or wind around neck.

Wristwatch

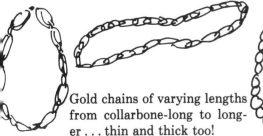

Gold chains of varying lengths from collarbone-long to longer . . . thin and thick too!

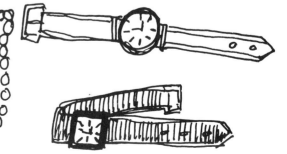

BASIC JEWELRY WARDROBE

EVENING

Ears

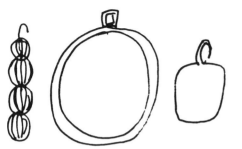

Larger important gold earring (hoops)

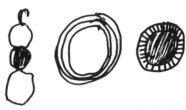

Semiprecious stones (mixed and single set in gold—larger, more important shapes)
Pearls set in gold (with or without sparkle)

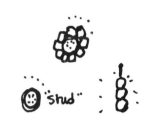

Diamonds set in gold (sparkle is important)

Necks

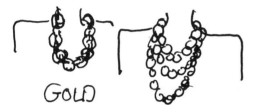

Gold—Heavier gold chains to wear in multiples plus one major gold necklace
Semiprecious stone necklaces to wear in multiples—always linked in gold metal.
Ropes mixed of pearls and gold and sparkle and colored stones.

Wrists

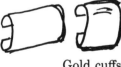

Gold cuffs

Inlayed gold and stones, bangles and cuffs

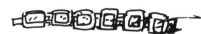

Sparkle and colored stones set in gold

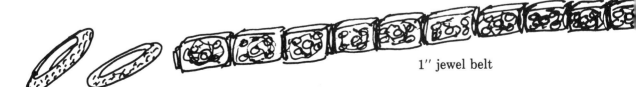

1″ jewel belt

Beaten gold bangles

- **TO COLLECT:** Necklaces of chunks or beads of semiprecious stones—all of one stone—or mixed: tiger-eye and carnelian with an occasional gold bead—or lapis lazuli and malachite, coral. Length should just skim the collarbone. Mix them and wear in multiples and with gold! Then collect longer rope versions.

- Wear one or two mineral necklaces or one with a gold chain. This can make all the difference in the look of a sweater or blouse. It can turn a look instantly from country to city (lunch/conference, etc.) pulled-together chic!
Wrists:

- *Classic watch*: The best every day watch as simple as possible! Think man's watch even if you choose a scaled-down version: round-faced (or square or oval), easy-to-read dial (white face, black numerals), leather strap, in brown leather or pigskin.

- Black leather only if you are clearly committed to black leather accessories for day.

- For sport/country: one with a metal flexible band that looks like a man's version is great, country-chic, and efficient-looking!

- For summer or hot places, a tan leather band.

Classic Bracelets

- Gold bangles in different widths. 2″ wide is the ideal day cuff width! Wear narrower ones in families of twos, threes, fours. Add a hefty chain link bracelet. Think again for proportion at least the thickness of a man's pocket-watch chain. If you can carry it, go wider or wear several. *Remember: doing up wrists and neck adds the dash and glamour to something so simple as a blouse and pair of trousers!*

- Classic Day Look: Wear watch and chain bracelet on same wrist. This is easy enough for a day in the country and a *pretty* touch!

- *Collect*: Cuffs and bangles of wood, wood inlayed with gold, wood inlayed with mother of pearl. Wood is more than basic *brown* color. There are shades that begin at almost washed-cream and go through tones of grayed taupe to peanut, walnut, cocoa, and chocolate. There are rosy fruitwoods, wood with a cast of deep crimson or burnt sienna to the almost black of ebony! Any of these look fabulous with gold and tones of gray, browns, or

navy for day. Any mix well with semiprecious stones and minerals (lapis, tiger-eye, carnelian, jade, etc.)

- *Collect*: bangles of ivory and bone (perfect for summer) and natural horn (plain or carved bangles). Wear one or two or mix one gold, one wood inlayed with gold, one narrow brown horn. Mix one ivory, two tones of wood, *one jade bangle, cinnabar from China* (which is crimson), jade and ebony wood! The trick is to build a collection of semiprecious and real materials: wood, horn, ivory, plus gold (real or not) jewelry. The pieces then become as interchangeable as tweed and gray flannel.

- *Play:* **Try combinations.** Add more. *Experiment.* Then study the result in a *full length mirror*, top to toe! Is the proportion perfect? Is there too much of an overload? If you are the *least* bit in question about the amount of jewelry you are wearing, *remove some. It is always better to have too little than too much.* No matter what, you must feel *perfectly* comfortable. *You must feel* beautiful! You must never feel *awkward or showy* (even at 8:30 A.M. on the bus to work). *This is one of the secrets of how to look your best!*

BASIC JEWELRY WARDROBE

• **Trick:** Try toning jewelry for day. With browns: wood, tortoise, horn, etc. Then use color in only one spot: a gold ear, a jade bangle slipped in with wood.... This is a sure way to avoid the look of too much jewelry. And it's very subtle and attractive.

Day

Earrings

Classic! Have at least two sizes of gold hoops—from a small, thin, almost-wire to something heftier. Collect them, as many sizes and versions as you can handle! This depends on your size, length of neck, etc. If you can carry the really huge "Duel in the Sun" kind, they can be an Instant Late-Day Look-maker. Slick your hair back and wear them with perfect makeup. They can turn a sweater-and-trouser look, or T-shirt and gauze skirt, into "alluring and sexy-terrific"!

• *Tip:* If you can afford it, it pays to try to collect *all* of these *basic gold pieces in real gold* (or gold-plated silver). Chances are they will be in your life forever even if you *don't* wear them for a season! They become an investment.

Classic: A Gold Stud Earring: Even if you don't have pierced ears, get the clip-on variety! There will often be the moment when you want a *bit* of light near your face without looking overly earring-y!—in the country or when you're wearing a chunky necklace, or when you don't feel like wearing jewelry but want a finish to your turnout! Begin to collect them from tiny-seed size to dime size.

• *Collect stud earrings in colors of minerals and semiprecious stones:* carnelian (orangey caramel color), blood coral (red), tigereye (gold/black/brown stone like a cat's eye), soft green jade, malachite (darker, brighter green), turquoise, lapis lazuli (deep cobalt blue), garnet, pearls. Studs of pale stones such as amethyst (mauve), pink quartz, moon-stone (almost clear milky), citrine (clear lemon), rock crystal. These pale colors look delicious in the daytime with pale silk. Even if you're wearing tweed and pale silk is your blouse. If you can afford them, collect the real kind. As they are semiprecious stones and minerals they can be surprisingly reasonable in price. Otherwise look for make-believe versions which can be amazingly real-looking!

• **Diamond studs** are handy and instantly attractive (especially if you have pierced ears, as there is less chance of losing them). The little bit of glisten and glitter is always a lift. Wear them *all day* no matter where, even at the beach!

• *The point of studs and small hoops:* They are a *nice* finish—a nice *complement*. They do what makeup does: give your face a lift, a lightness. They are not overpowering.

• Note: Do the same with *Silver* as with *Gold*. Collect studs, especially if you particularly like the look of silver. Pretty silver hoops in summer are a super look! Think of them with *silver* sandals, *silver* bangles. Mixing metal takes a knack, so match if you don't want to risk looking mismatched.

Necklaces

Classic: Chains of gold. Slightly hefty ones. Think the weight or size of a man's pocket-watch chain for proportion—one, two, or three.
• Length: Chains should just edge under collarbone. This is a good length for most necklaces. It is a neck-lengthener and doesn't risk looking droopy or draggy!

• **Extra-fine gold chains:** you can wear an extra-fine gold chain forever without it being noticed. Many women do just that—they *add* jewelry over it! Remember, fine gold chains don't count for much when one is speaking "jewelry." They look nice with a bathing suit on the beach—a tiny glistening in the sun—and sexy in the bathtub.

Evening

• Nighttime earrings want to be more *important*. Just how large depends on (1) your proportion: hair length, neck length, and (2) what you are wearing. Study the look in a *full-length* mirror. Those small counter mirrors in stores tell you nothing except how the earring looks near your skin. *You can only judge proportion by seeing yourself head-to-toe!*

• **Gold!** You have already begun a collection of gold pieces—jewelry, a belt, sandals, etc. *A major gold earring and some gold bracelets plus a gold belt and gold sandals are the magic trick to make a day look into instant evening!*

• Drop earrings are wonderful, but depending again on proportion, hair lengths, neck length, etc. They can make you look draggy if too big.

• **Sparkle!** Diamonds, ruby-colored and emerald and sapphire-colored stones mixed together or singly. Sparkle mixed with semiprecious stones: diamonds and onyx

(shiny black) look wonderful with a slide-of-black bare dress for night! "Emeralds" mixed with caramelly carnelian, "ruby" and lapis lazulis are instant Evening Look-Makers!

• **Tip:** *Make sure that all sparkle is set in gold.* This way no matter what other metal piece you add (i.e., cuffs) there won't be a clash.

• **Semiprecious stone** earrings (real or copies!) mixed together and/or with gold. Again these are as handy and magic as big gold ears. Always make sure the metal is *gold-colored!*

NECKS: Build on day. Wear three or four gold-link chains. *Add* one string of coral chunks—fabulous with all-black or all-white! Wear plain gold ears and some gold bracelets.

• *Or build a neck of three necklaces,* chunks of amethyst, or three strings of carved citrine—pale lemon color and smashing with ivory, especially if you are a little tanned. Or one onyx and gold necklace plus two of chunks of coral. Or wear one important gold necklace. As with major earrings, this *alone* can be the magic evening touch!

• **Remember:** *Balance!* Unclutter! If you are wearing ma-

jor earrings you will probably want to skip a necklace—only add bracelets. If you are wearing a major necklace you will want only the *smallest* stud earrings chosen from day group for a bit of light at your face—an arm of glorious bracelets, no necklace, and medium-sized earrings and *always* perfect hands, makeup and hair—*balance!*

WRISTS: A pair of *gold cuffs,* the ultra-easy evening magic maker. You don't have to think. When you want to change a day sweater (or blouse) and pants to evening quickly, kick off your shoes, slip on your gold sandals, *put on your gold cuffs.* Their width depends on your size and proportion. 1-½'' to 2'' is a good median!

• *Handy evening bracelets:* Gold-and-stone inlayed cuffs and bangles. Add these to your day collection: two jade bangles plus a wider cuff of jade and carnelian. Play!

• *Hammered gold bangles* (or earrings) are wonderful to own for evening. The hammering creates light-catching facets which glint prettily in night light—great for restaurants in low light where gestures are so important.

• *Discover: If you find a beautiful jeweled belt that*

works for your proportion, buy it! Like gold cuffs it's a *magic-maker*. Slip it on with black sweater and pants, a dark silky dress, or one of black wool jersey—even with jeans and a beautiful satiny shirt for country evenings. It can be the glorious Chanel kind that is burnished gold links with a filigree buckle, gold metal over-studded with stones, or, if *you have a silver collection* (ears, sandals, bangles) silver studded with turquoise or coral, or a narrow flat chain belt of mixed gold-and-silver-colored metal. **Key:** *It must look like a treasure even if it is not real*; otherwise it could work bad magic and look cheap.

• **Accessorizing rule:** *Don't forget the full-length mirror top-to-toe.* Study the proportion. Play! Experiment! Then check it before going out the door.

• **Accessory rule:** If even a hint of "overload," unload! *Better too little than too much.*

• *Trick*: As you do for day, try *toning jewelry for night.* This is a safe way to begin! Using accessories, jewelry, etc., takes practice. It takes *ease of handling.* Accessories of any kind must look effortless as if they are meant to be! *Toning example*: if you're wearing pale beige silk, wear ivory or pale stone colors at wrists and neck and only one "hit" of gold at ears. Or wear all black with jewelry of black onyx and dark spinach jade. Add one *slice* of a gold bracelet with the dark stone colors!

• **Un-accessory:** *Sometimes it looks wonderful to wear practically no jewelry at night*: a pale printed peachy georgette blouse, taupe silk pajamas, gold sandals, gold belt—*no bracelets.* The georgette edges of cuffs are beautiful and delicate alone, but *make certain your hands are perfect!* Wear nothing at your neck. The neckline curve of the blouse is enough with just skin. Wear only the tiniest gold-and-diamond at ear for a glint of light near your face only. Perfect hair and makeup ultra-important! *Fragile and delicate is beautiful!* You might tuck a fresh full-blown peach rose in your belt or in your hair.

• *Accessory Tip:* EXPERIMENT. Don't be afraid to play! Build necks, build wrists for day looks and evening looks! *On a quiet afternoon put all your jewelry out on your bed.* See what combinations you can invent. *Mix* textures, combinations, all toned pieces with one slash of color or shine. All shine and one slice of color, combinations of three colors, two colors plus shine, etc. Put ears, wrists, and necks together. *Make up recipes*. Write them down, if you like, as a memory aid! Try them on. This way you begin to know how to *use* your collection. This not only saves time but allows for surprise inventions of more ways to use what you own, and most importantly you learn ease of handling! *Being comfortable, looking as if it's effortless is the key to it all.*

• *Remember:* For day and evening, unclutter and balance. **Remember**; tone jewelry. If you are not certain, play it safe. You can wear more this way without looking like a Christmas tree!

• *Evening trick*: A *fresh flower.* Tuck one into a silky shirt neckline, opened as low

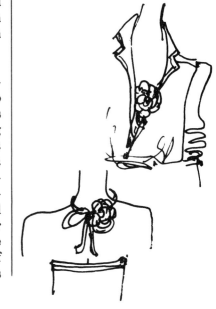

as possible, into the side of a narrow necklace. Wear one at your neck with a narrow cord of satin tied in a bow (charming do-it-yourself necklace!). Bow-knot the cord as high or low as you need for neck length. Slip the flower stem into the knot *before* "bowing" to keep flower secure. Tuck a flower into a narrow bracelet cuff to wear at wrist as a Summer Touch.

• *NOTE ON PINS*: They are handy day and evening enhancers, that "nice touch." Collect them to play with instead of a necklace: a pretty gold metal one pinned high to the collar of a turtleneck or cowl sweater. Pin a pale stone-and-gold one to the knot of an asymmetrically worn chiffon scarf at night. Pin a carved wood one to a cotton scarf for summer day. A gold-and-silver

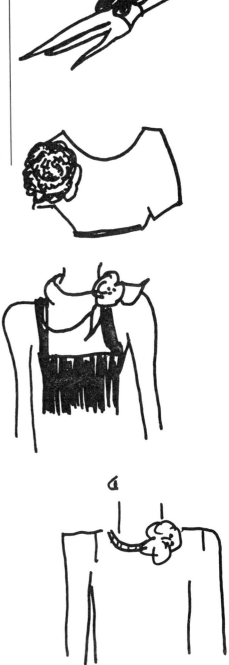

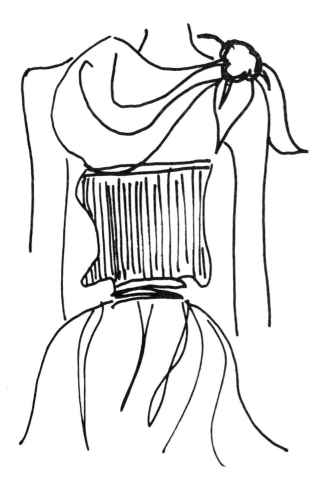

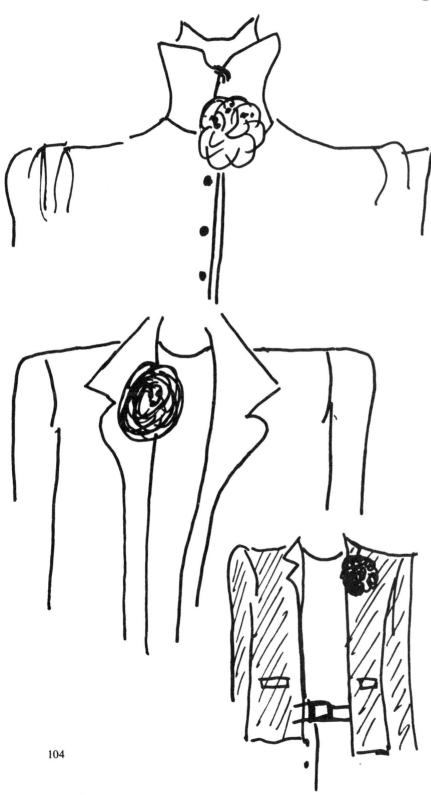

pin to the edge of the round curve of a cardigan sweater or T-shirt, or a wonderful gold or combination gold-and-tigereye to the lapel of a jacket or coat! All these are great-looking touches. Use a "flower" pin of coral or carved ivory or a carved rectangle of jade to hold collar of a silk blouse closed and change the look of an open collar.

• **Pin a *real* flower** to the lapel of a jacket—tweed jacket, plus sweater and trousers and a small gardenia in the lapel—a surprise and a lovely feminine touch! Try pinning a pale pink camellia on a white linen suit.

Tip: JEWELRY FOR SUMMER OR HOT PLACES. Keep it light and cool! Pale materials—bone, shell, ivory, mother of pearl, woven straw, pale tones of wood, pale stone colors, etc. *Use metal sparingly.* Big cuffs of gold or silver can look and feel too hot. That is not to deny the magic of big gold hoops or the smashing look of one cuff of carved silver studded with coral to wear with gauzy black cotton at night, but an overload on a 90° day looks (and feels) too much!

Tips on Jewelry

• Wash metal in warm soapy water. Polish with cream (depending on kind of metal). Buff with a soft cloth.

• Keep metal pieces separated—earrings, rings, bracelets, etc.—in small flannel bags to cut down on scratching and tarnishing or wrap pieces in squares of flannel bought by the yard and then place in plastic zip-lock bags (to hold them by groups).

• *Real tortoiseshell and horn*: keep away from heat and light. Polish from time to time with olive oil. They tend to dry out. If you live in a steam-heated house or dry climate, be sure to keep an open container of water nearby to minimize checking (tiny cracks) and warping! If you need to do this, store pieces on a closed shelf or in a cabinet so that you can keep them near their water supply safely and insure a close, moist atmosphere.

• *Ivory*: Wash with mild soap (never detergent) and warm water. Give pieces an occasional "massage" with baby oil. Remove excess with a soft tissue. Sometimes a bath in milk can help remove discolorations. Remember, ivory is porous. It tends to dry out in extreme dry-climate conditions. As with tortoise shell, keep close to an open container of water in a *closed* shelf or cabinet so that the atmosphere remains moist.

• AMBER: Wash in warm, soapy water (never detergent). Massage with oil from time to time to keep lustrous.

• NEVER scrub any jewelry of set stones with a toothbrush, ammonia, detergent. *Never* boil in a pot. Scrubbing tends to loosen settings, and harsh chemicals can eat at the surface of the stones. Boiling is too harsh and shocking! To clean, soak them in *warm*, pure soapy water. Dry well with a hair dryer so that no moisture remains in any crevice.

• *For safety, have expensive jewelry, real materials, gems, and semiprecious stones professionally cleaned.*

• Remember that extreme temperature change can crack stones and alter their color. Coral, jade, and tigereye are all temperature sensitive and shock sensitive. Don't drop! Handle like fine china. They, too, can break or chip easily.

• Tip: Remove all jewelry before cleaning house, gardening, etc.

• Be sure to examine bead-stringing of necklaces and bracelets carefully from time to time. Threads soil, stretch, and wear from the constant weight of beads. Restring before they have a chance to break. Always have round

beads strung between knots and use silk. Nylon is too stiff, so beads never hang beautifully. This goes especially for pearls!

• *Wearing is good for pearls.* Body oils keep them alive! Never store in bags; they need air to breathe.

TIP: A LOVELY WAY TO STORE JEWELRY—If you have the space, it looks wonderful to keep your treasures in the open on a dresser, wood table, marble-topped cabinet in your bedroom or bathroom. Not only can you enjoy looking at them, but also it keeps you from forgetting what you own; i.e., those coral studs that you bought in Hawaii two years ago! *Fill small baskets or pretty paper boxes or tiny china dishes*: one for earhoops, one for studs, one for gold chains, one for pins . . . a wicker tray filled with bracelets! Or use antique glass salt cellars that have been forever in your kitchen cabinet, individual china ashtrays for the dinner table, little silver "nut" dishes, small silver trays, all those totally impractical, unused gifts (grandmother's inheritance, wedding presents, etc.). Check the back shelves of your china cabinet! All these make terrific holders for your jewelry collection.

BASIC SCARF——
WARDROBE

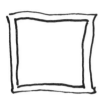

24″ squares

silk crepe de chine
cotton

all colors
solids and *small* checks
prints
stripes

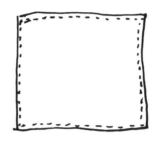

30″–36″ squares

silk crepe de chine
cotton
silk twill
silk and wool
thinnest wool

all colors
solids and small checks
prints
stripes

Muffler

silk twill (like a man's)
silk crepe de chine
silk and wool
cashmere (like a man's)
knit

all colors
solids
stripes
in thin silk, small prints

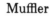

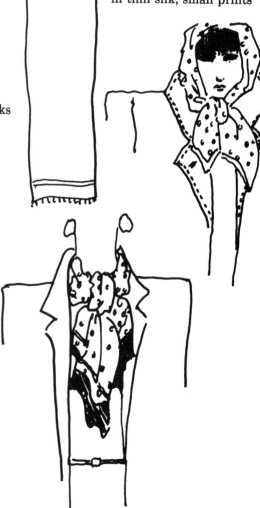

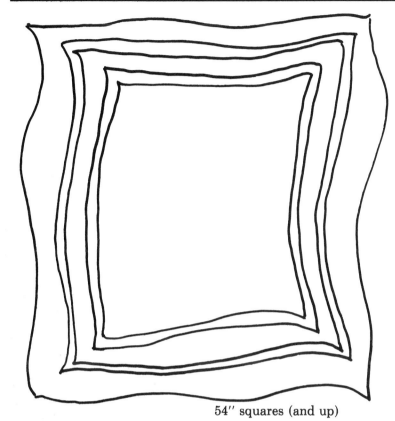

54″ squares (and up)

(Shawl, sarong, blanket)
silk crepe de chine
georgette/chiffon (*silk*)
thin cotton & cotton gauze
cashmere
knitted cashmere/wool
alpaca/wool
soft wool

all colors
plaids
(alpaca/wool, soft wool)
larger & large prints
(silk, cotton, georgette)

On the following pages you will find the complete story: squares and oblongs of fabric from silk to cotton to knitted cashmere to lambswool. These can be the most versatile and useful things you own!

Caution: Some of the looks may not be for you, depending on your figure problems. Stay away from hip-sarongs if you are hip/derriere-heavy. Omit bosom-tying if you are overly bosomy unless you devise your own invention using a perfect strapless bra underneath! *But* wrapping into "shawls" is a boon to large figures, big hips, etc. This can be attractive camouflage!

Remember: Wearing scarves and shawls takes practice. You must have the will. The negative "I'm all thumbs" approach will not work! Play with them in front of a full-length mirror on a rainy afternoon. You will discover you can master any of these looks!

Tricks With Scarves

• **Tip: Experiment!** The knack of wearing scarves well comes from being able to handle them. This takes practice. All fabrics move differently, respond differently. One day when *you* have time take a stack of scarves that you already own. As many different sizes and materials as possible —cotton, silk, wool, chiffon, etc! Sit in front of a mirror and play. Knot them. See how easily or bulkily they knot, how they drape around your shoulders, how some puff up and look stiff, how others hang limp, how some sizes do just what you want and others feel unwieldy!

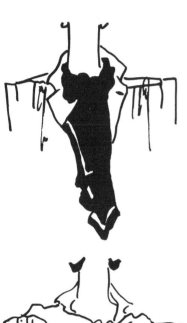

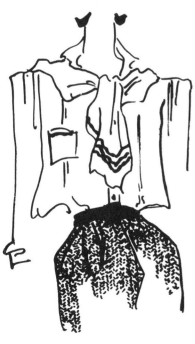

• *Practice the different suggestions listed below.* This is key! Once you begin to play stand back and *look at the whole effect top-to-toe.* Can you take the proportion? Do you look choked or top-heavy? Do you look longer and slimmer and is the whole effect uplifting? That, of course, is the goal. The only way a scarf or any accessory looks good is if it looks *effortless*, natural, and *wonderful*. Otherwise take it off!

Tip: Fabric and size are key. The fabric must be soft and tyable . . . silky, gauzy or thin knit . . . Again, remember before you buy any scarf (or fabric by the yard to make a scarf), hold it up by a corner and watch how it falls. Tie two ends to see if it ties magically or if the knot becomes a tennis ball!
Size Guide:
Squares
12″ Man's handkerchief size: to short-knot, to tie up collars
15″–24″ Neck wraps, headband wraps
27″–30″ Waist wraps, head wraps
36″–45″ Shoulder wraps, head wraps (babushkas, etc.)
54″–60″ Shawls and sarongs

Oblongs: Mufflers, waist ties (only if very thin, i.e. chiffon! or cotton gauze).
45″ × 51″ sarong length: skirts, etc.

Note: 60″ wide fabric by the yard (51″ long) will make the perfect bosom to ankle-long "sarong" for beach or evening! All you have to do is machine-stitch or hand-roll the edges as narrowly as possible.
45″ × 100″ "Serape" length: To wear as a shawl, blanket

The Scarf Wardrobe Essentials

• **Collect:** Squares of silk (24″, 30″, 36″) to tie in neck of blouses, coats, dresses. Remember, the shorter your neck or the bigger your bosom, the less you want to muffle. Wear smaller, neater, toned-to-top ones and TIE LOW!

• **Collect:** Big 54″ squares of silk to use as shawls in the summer or at night.

• **Collect:** Mufflers of silk, knitted cashmere or lambswool (like a man's muffler) to slide under the collar of a coat or jacket, especially in cool weather. Ideal length: When you hang it around your neck, ends should be no longer than top-of-hipbone; otherwise mufflers look unwieldy and too droopy.

• *Remember, the shorter you are and the longer you want to look, the shorter the muffler!*

• **Collect:** Squares of *cotton* for summer or warm places—

24″, 30″, 36″—to tie at the neck, on your head, to use as waist-ties. 54″ ones to use as shawls or sarongs on the beach.

• REMEMBER: *COLOR!* Here is where you *collect color*—the rainbow! Scarves are the color dash to your wardrobe. They last *forever,* so count on adding and adding!

• **Collect** *SOLIDS AND PRINTS.* Small men's wear tie designs on silk always look super for city/business day. Find little flowers, checks on silk and cotton for summer, wonderful stripes. Save huge flowers and large prints for big 54″ squares.

RULE: *The smaller the scarf, the smaller the pattern.* If you stick to this you will always love your collection and rarely tire of it!

• Be sure to look for hand-rolled or machine hand-rolled edges. If fringed the fringes should be at least 1½″ deep on silk—deeper on wool. The finish of scarves is key.

• *Buy the best*! Scarves are the prime example of investment; *they work forever.* They are clearly timeless! Beautiful silk, crepe de chine, and cashmere will always perform superbly *and* always make what you are wearing look more expensive!

Basic Ways To Wear a Scarf

• On folding scarves: For neck-tying and waist-tying *always fold in thirds.* The scarf becomes less bulky and holds and wraps the body better since you are using the bias of the fabric to tie.

• Tied loosely *inside* a collar: The more neck length you need the lower you tie. The shorter you are, the smaller the square . . . Try 24″ instead of 30″ or 36,″ especially if it is not toned to your top!

• Tie *under* a collar, Girl Scout fashion. This is particularly good to do if you want to use a scarf *and* you've a short neck. It shows the maximum skin! *Do not do this tie if you have big bosoms.* The bulk of the scarf hits exactly where you do not want bulk!

• Hang a silky or wool muffler (or 36″ square folded diagonally—point under collar at back) loosely under a collar. This is best to do with a jacket, coat, dress. Make sure that ends of the muffler don't hang lower than the top of hipbone—otherwise, too draggy. Tone muffler to what you're wearing if you have big bosoms. **Proportion note:** If you are heavy, wearing a scarf this way is a good trick. Drawing the eye "inward"—away from the

sides of the body, it's a width-minimizer, but no horizontal or big patterns, please! *Wear a muffler this way* if you want broad shoulders to look less *broad.* Make sure if the fabric is a pattern that it runs *vertically,* never horizontally!

• A pretty way to "fill" the neckline of a crewneck sweater is to wrap a scarf at your neck. (Lower as you need to for length.) Tone it to what you're wearing, i.e., navy sweater and trousers, brown belt, navy silk scarf with a *fine* line of red running through. Or make it your "slash" of color: navy sweater and trousers, brown belt, *bordeaux* silk scarf. The *trick* is to keep it from looking "unbulky," twist it before you wrap it around!

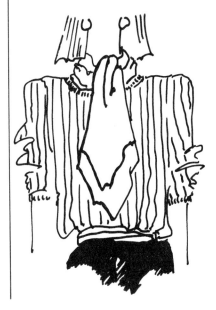

BASIC SCARF WARDROBE

TRICK: Try pinning a pretty pin to overlap.

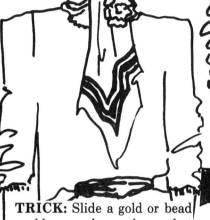

TRICK: Slide a gold or bead necklace underneath so that just a bit of gold peeks through between scarf and neckline.

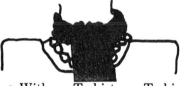

• With a T-shirt or T-shirt dress, *wrap and twist* a short cotton scarf at the neck. Hold closed with a *wood pin* or one of bright red or cobalt blue lacquer for evening. It is the way to "turn" a T-shirt into a finished look!

Day: bordeaux T-shirt, navy cotton pants or skirt, small navy cotton scarf twisted at neck and pinned with walnut-colored pin. Add tan leather belt and sandals, one or two wood bangles, perhaps a small gold hoop earring, and you've a city/day look!

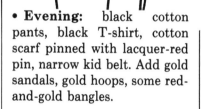

• **Evening:** black cotton pants, black T-shirt, cotton scarf pinned with lacquer-red pin, narrow kid belt. Add gold sandals, gold hoops, some red-and-gold bangles.

• *If you have a long neck*, a nice way to wear a small cotton scarf with a bare top: Twist it tightly. Wrap your neck and *knot the scarf in back*. Looks great with hair slicked back into a small knot or neat pony tail! Make sure scarf ends are

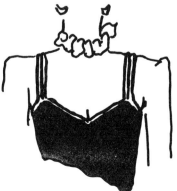

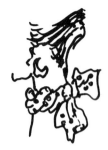

short after you knot; otherwise wrap once again around neck and knot in front. You see why you need a lot of neck for this!

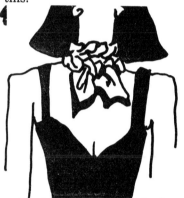

• Another bare-top trick that shows skin and is not neck-binding . . . try it! Tie and knot a beautiful 36″ square scarf *fichu-style*—your prettiest silk one (perhaps a pale peach color to wear with a cream camisole top dress!) Tie it loosely and *asymmetrically* over shoulders. A lovely summer evening trick that keeps the air-conditioning chill off! You can adjust it to keep your neck longest. When you slide it asymmetrically, flip one scarf end over one shoulder; this helps keep the scarf balanced and in place.

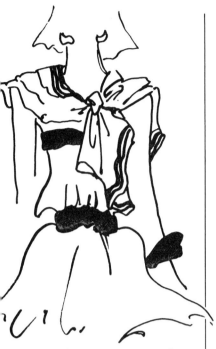

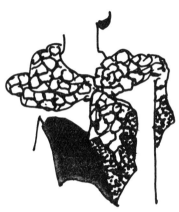

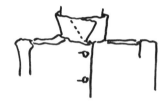

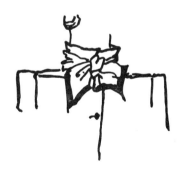

• **Scarf trick** with a soft blouse if you have the neck length: Stand the collar of your blouse up. This is prettiest to do with a silk blouse and *especially* one without a collar stand. Wrap one end over the other so that it stands high around your neck, then wrap a silk scarf around it (high like a stock) to hold it all in place.

• Instead of knotting, just loop one end over the other and adjust the whole scarf so that it falls softly and beautifully over your shoulders a *little* asymmetrically so you don't look too "Martha Washington"! This is best to do when you are bare shouldered (no sleeves) *and* with a scarf as delicate and floaty as possible, i.e., thin chiffon or thinnest cotton gauze! *Variations:* For a romantic touch, tuck a fresh flower into the knot! Or pin a pretty pin through a part of the knot and through the shoulder strap of your bare top. This looks pretty and also holds fichu in place! Be sure you pin carefully so that nothing pulls out of kilter and the scarf falls nicely.

Trick: For an easy-to-wear SLASH OF COLOR fling a square of silk folded diagonally over one shoulder. Use silk crepe de chine or chiffon if possible—they fall wonderfully. This looks casual and dashing, especially in summer or at night. *The bigger the square, the better, and no smaller than a 36" square or it will look skimpy!* A magenta scarf over a black T-shirt. A bright yellow one over a white sweater and pants, or a pale pink over bare shoulders with a navy strapless camisole and skirt!

BASIC SCARF WARDROBE

This is also nice to do with a man's small silk pocket handkerchief! It is just long enough to knot in a short, perky knot in front. A navy silk blouse "tied up" with a navy silk square with white pin dots . . . A cream blouse "tied up" with a small square of cream with black dots . . . A brown one with brown silk paisley print. Remember: the smaller the scarf the snappier (therefore the pocket handkerchief). However, if you can take the proportion, you *can* do it with a larger scarf. Wrap front to back and front again. Knot in front. (As romantic as Lord Byron!)

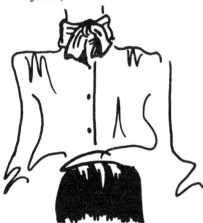

• *Variation*: Wrap blouse collar and tie it in with a bow in front with 4″ wide black satin ribbon. It looks wonderful on a white or cream blouse worn at night with black trousers, black gold-edged belt, and gold sandals. *Remember, you must have the neck length to do this.*

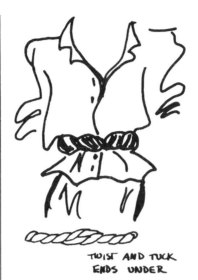

TWIST AND TUCK
ENDS UNDER

• **Scarf as waist wrap— sensational** summer belt. A great way to change the look of a solid silk shirtdress: wrap the waist with a narrow-striped scarf, one color of which being the color of the dress. **For dash**, unbutton the dress to the waist and wear a bare cotton camisole underneath. **Tip:** by twisting the striped scarf, you get an interesting diagonal play of lines!

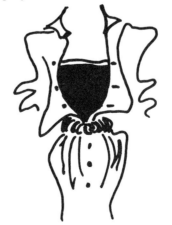

• **Scarf "Necklace":** loop a small *oblong* of silk at your neck. Wear it over "skin" with a thin, loose silk or handkerchief-cotton jacket. Be sure to keep scarf a lovely skin-flattering color. A nice variation instead of a necklace, especial-

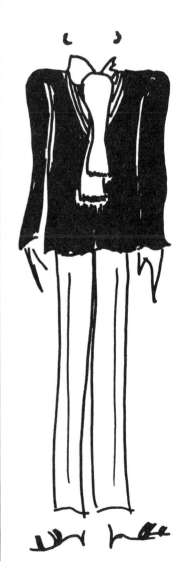

ly for summer night. *Pretty color is key!* Try a white silk man's evening muffler! It is a super look with a thin black cotton pajama jacket, matching pants, bright red or green sandals, black lacquer bangles, one gold bangle, and gold hoop earrings!

HAIR TRICKS: Scarves create instant hair looks. A small square (18″ or 24″) of silk or cotton twisted tightly (to make a narrow "snake") and tied in hair instead of a ribbon—or twisted and wrapped like a wide hairband—or folded diagonally and wrapped in a small neat turban (a 30″ square). These are all especially nice in summer—so airy and fresh and cool to slick hair back and wrap color into it! *For winter*, there is no better head protector than a scarf of wool or knitted cashmere!

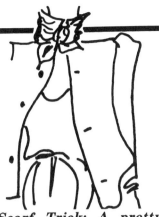

• *Scarf Trick: A pretty way to make a soft blouse into an instant jacket.* Tie the blouse at the neck with a small square of silk or short oblong silk scarf. Try to match or tone the scarf to the color of the blouse. Wear the blouse open from the neck down *as a jacket* over a bare camisole for evenings or over a sweater and skirt for day, i.e., a red silk blouse, knotted at neck with dark red square of silk over brown sweater and skirt. This is a very pretty way to use a blouse/scarf combination as a "hit of color"!

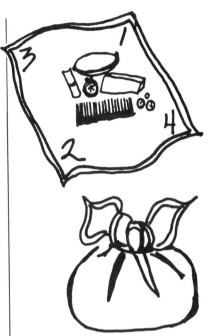

TRICK: A SCARF IS AN INSTANT HANDBAG! (12″, 24″, 36″ squares) Pile your essentials in the center of the square and knot like a knapsack. *A weekend bag*: 54″ square. *For evening*: little squares of silk or satin. *Day country*: 36″ square of flowered chintz. *"Suitcase" for a summer country weekend*: Take a huge square of cotton (a piece of batik, or an Indian cotton block-printed table cloth), fold all your weekend clothes and pile them in the center of square. Knot ends diagonally to each other as you sometimes do with laundry piled in a sheet! Then make it into a shoulder bag: After you knot everything securely, take the two opposite long ends and knot again, this time towards

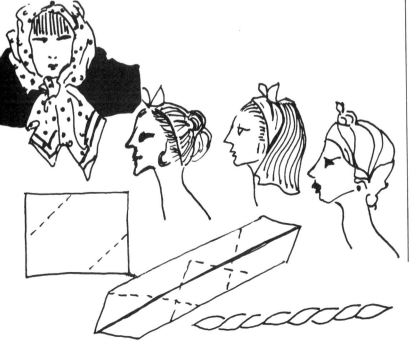

the ends. This creates a sling-loop which you then slide over your shoulder. It looks wonderful in "hot places"!

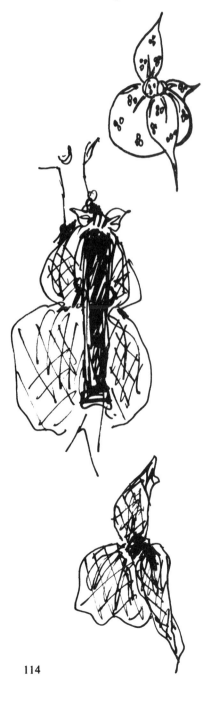

TRICK: Instant Necklace: Take one 12″ square (one of thin satin or printed silk) and fold in thirds on bias. Knot in the center. Stand up the collar of your blouse. Place the knot at center front of collar and tie in back in a short knot. Or, variation: Take a 24″ square of pretty silk print, satin, or *thin* cotton. Fold in thirds on bias. Knot *several* times and do the same.

• *A new take on a belt*: A 36″ square this time, folded and knotted (as the neck version) and short-knotted in back of waist. Note: keep knots close together (1″–1½″ spaced). Make sure they stay in center front and don't end up at *sides* of waist to make waist look thick. Pretty to wear with a T-shirt dress or a T-shirt and trousers.

• **Collect 54″ (or larger) squares** of knitted cashmere or lambswool or a *thin* square blanket of woven alpaca and wool (solid, striped or plaid). Add for evening and warm places: *54″ squares of amazing colors and patterns of silk with self-fringed edges.* These "perfect pieces" are compatible with any type and length of dressing from jeans and a sweater to day dresses to jackets and pants to long evening wear—they are a perfect proportion and finish always!

How to wear a blanket/shawl

• Wear it *over a coat* as an *added layer of warmth.* Muffle into it, wrap it around when you need protection . . . wear it slung over one shoulder (very dashing!) when you don't need protection! A camel-colored coat, brown tweed skirt, brown and cocoa *knitted blanket shawl*, brown stockings and flat shoes, brown leather shoulder bag make an attractive easy city/suburban town turnout!

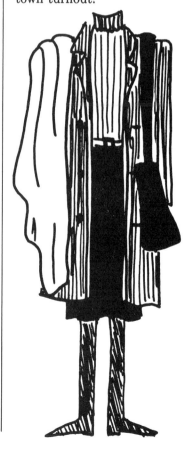

• Wear *the blanket shawl the same way over a jacket!* This is a great look *and* it serves as a "coat" when you need it. A navy suit, vicuña-colored sweater, vicuña-knitted cashmere shawl, dark peanut leather belt, shoes, stockings toned to shoe color for a terrific city look!

• *A blanket shawl can turn a sweater (or blouse) and trousers (or skirt) into a finished look*: Cream silk blouse, navy skirt, navy-and-vicuña cashmere shawl . . . or navy trousers, ivory sweater, navy, cream-and-vicuña-striped alpaca and wool square (folded as a giant triangle) over one shoulder. The blanket shawl does the same as a jacket. *It pulls the look together!*

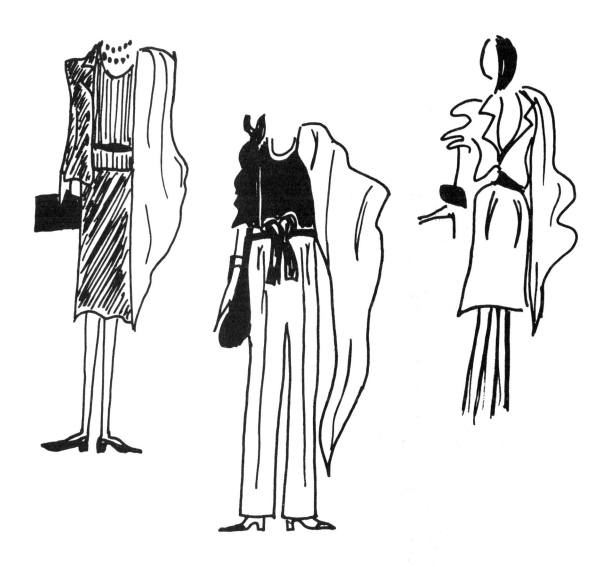

BASIC SCARF WARDROBE

• The same navy, vicuña, and cream shawl as a *late-day covering* with a bare navy silk camisole and skirt. Add black satin ribbon bowed at the waist, black satin sandals!

• A blanket shawl as *evening cover* for pajama dressing or long "important" dress dressing: pale gray jacquarded-satin tunic, pajama, black cashmere knit blanket shawl, dark silver sandals, belt, tiny bag. *Evening:* Dark rose chiffon long evening dress, black cashmere blanket shawl, dark silver slippers, with dark silver ribbon bowed at waist.

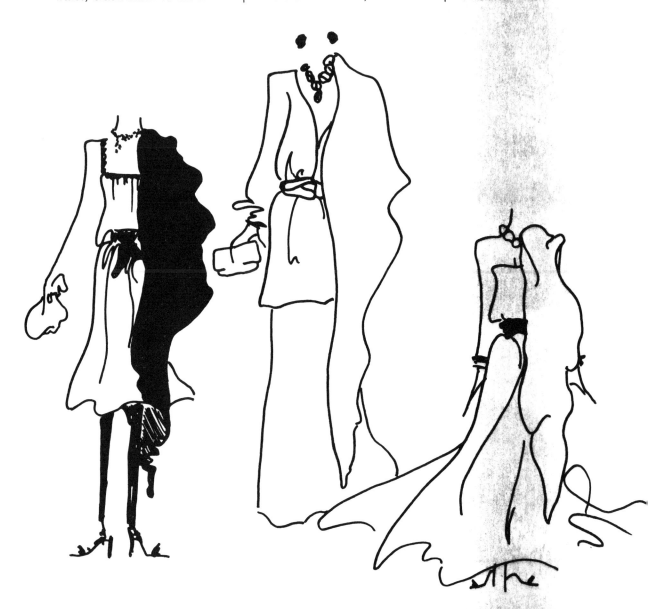

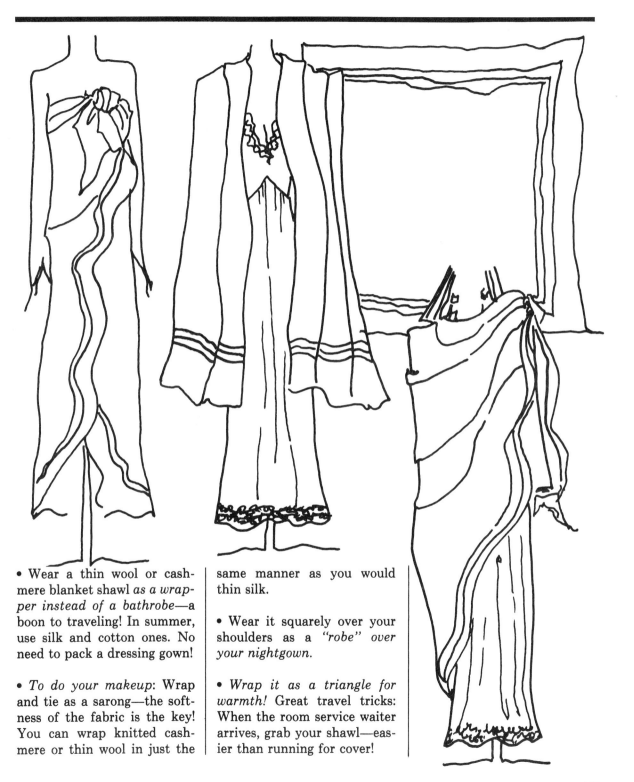

• Wear a thin wool or cash-mere blanket shawl *as a wrapper instead of a bathrobe*—a boon to traveling! In summer, use silk and cotton ones. No need to pack a dressing gown!

• *To do your makeup*: Wrap and tie as a sarong—the soft-ness of the fabric is the key! You can wrap knitted cash-mere or thin wool in just the same manner as you would thin silk.

• Wear it squarely over your shoulders as a *"robe" over your nightgown.*

• *Wrap it as a triangle for warmth!* Great travel tricks: When the room service waiter arrives, grab your shawl—eas-ier than running for cover!

BASIC SCARF WARDROBE

• *A nice turn on a bed jacket for breakfast*—especially in bed. Fling your shawl over your shoulders. It is easy to move among pillows, bed covers, and breakfast tray.

• *Great for bed-reading* before lights-out: Wrap a shawl around your shoulders to take the chill off. When you go to sleep, it *can become an additional blanket.*

• *Travel Treasure*! Wear a shawl over your shoulder on a plane, in a car, etc. Wrap it as a proper blanket when you take a nap!

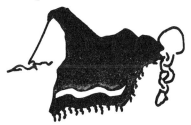

• **When you are not using your shawls,** (1) store in stacks in a pretty wicker trunk, (2) fold over antique quilt racks, (3) fold over the back of a chair (Your scarlet wool one could even add dash to the look of your living room.), or cover your bed with one!

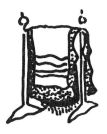

How To Do a Summer Weekend With a Stack of Scarves!

• **The "suitcase"**: A 45″ or 54″ square tied like a giant knapsack.

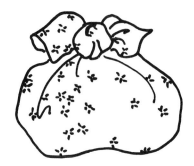

• **The scarf sizes you need:**
24″ squares For necks and head "bands"
27″ squares For head-ties, "bras," waist-ties
54″ squares For sarongs, skirts, "dresses"
45″ × 51″ Sarong lengths

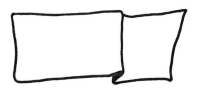

The fabrics: cotton and silk both printed and solid. Indian sari silk. These can be ready-made scarves, cotton gauze, and "shawls" or cotton and/or silk or lengths bought by the yard in fabric stores. **Tip:** For wonderful Indonesian batiks and Indian block print cotton (which look so amazing in the sun!), **find ethnic shops that specialize in oriental or Far Eastern goods or shops which sell Indian saris. For another wonderful sun look,** use lengths of cotton from Provence in Southern France (brightly colored block-printed flowers and paisleys). **Tip:** To find the right lengths for skirts, both short and ankle-length (and anywhere in between), check fabric widths. 45″ fabric = skirt (waist to knee) or *mini* "dress." 54″ means longer. 60″ means to the ankle! Hold them up to you and estimate.

• **Add to scarves:** T-shirts both bare and covered, a cotton shirt, silk blouse, one pair of thin cotton trousers, a silky or gauzy skirt, a bikini. Tone and play the colors so that everything works together!

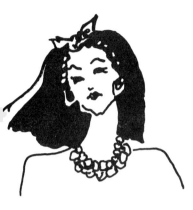

HEAD WRAPS

• Use bright cotton—printed or solid—**or white at the beach!** to twist and short-knot a "head-band" of a 24″ scarf.

• *Trick for beach hair:* Wet hair, slick back. Wet scarf and twist, then knot in hair. It's extra cool! Headwrap: 36″ cotton square (or 27″ for a smaller effect if you prefer) folded *on the bias*, gathered into a few front tucks and wrapped low on forehead. Knot the pointed end and secure knot at nape of neck. Ends are then left to fly free. **Trick:** to hold tucks in place while tying, pull ends taut after establishing the amount of tucks. Keep taut as you wrap and knot! Great for high-sun protection (or when you want to hide your hair)! Pulling low almost to brow is nicely mysterious.

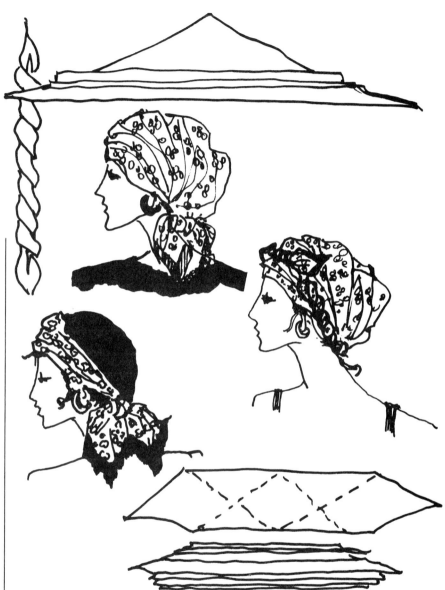

• Option: Instead of leaving ends free, after knotting securely at nape of neck, twist ends and wrap them around, running them just behind ears, to knot in a short-knot at top of head. Tuck in excess ends.

• Version #2: Fold a 27″ or 36″ scarf in thirds and "tucks." Pull taut and tie a *wide headband* as high or low on brow as you like. Again, you can leave ends free or twist and tie them at top of head.

119

BASIC SCARF WARDROBE

This wide headband works well with hair pulled sleek into a knot or ponytail. A nice look for drinks on a boat, at the beach club at end of day, etc. In any case, leave ears free—not covered—for a prettier line. Add gold hoops for more allure!

• *Scarf bra:* (1) Take a 27″ silk or cotton scarf, (2) fold in thirds, (3) knot in center, (4) with knot between breasts, arrange fullness where you need it and knot it back.

• Or do the reverse: (1) Fold scarf, (2) twist once tightly in center, instead of knotting, (3) with twist at center back bring ends forward, arrange fullness, and knot *in front* between breasts. The twist keeps the back part of scarf nicely narrow.

• *Halter:* You can do the same front knot with a *36″* scarf. Twist long ends, tie around neck.

• **Bicolored bra:** (1) Take two 24″ or 18″ squares.—A red and a black, rose and tan, or two tones of white. (2) Knot ends to each other in a *short knot*. (3) Fold excess. (4) Place knot between breasts. Pull and arrange over breasts. Knot in back. Tuck extra knot tails too long to hang free in sides. Lovely at night with *silk squares*. Wear with cotton or silk pants, a gauzy or silky skirt. Slide a shawl or a blouse/jacket on top!

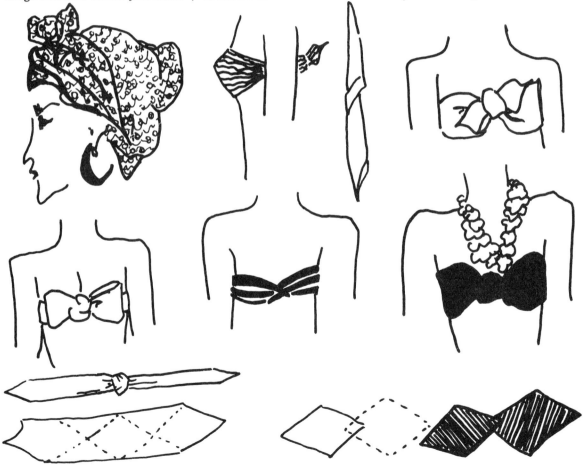

120

• **Wear as bikini top:** Pretty to do instead of wearing your matching bikini top, i.e., black bikini bottom, a scarf-bra of black ground-flowered cotton; white bikini bottom with a bright brilliant-pink scarf top. Wear with shorts, a skirt, or cotton pants underneath a pretty cotton or silky shirt or a thin jacket. A nice hot-day way to shop, go to lunch, etc.

• **Wear a scarf-bra as sexy evening look:** black silk scarf bra, red-flowered cotton skirt to calf, red sandals, a big 54″ black-and-red-cotton square as shawl thrown over your shoulder . . . Sensational!

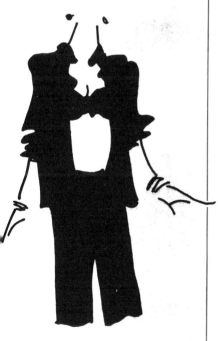

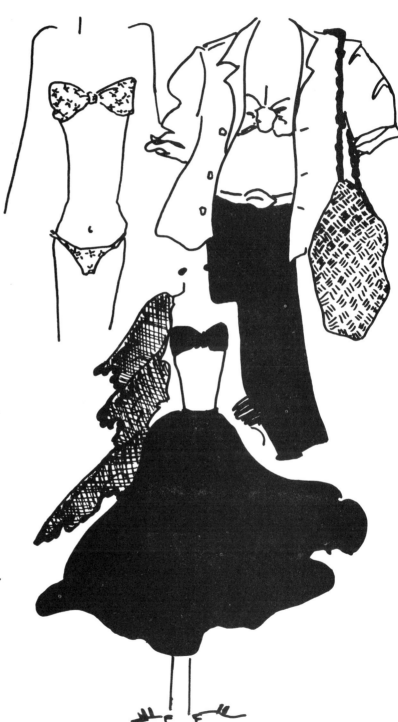

BASIC SCARF WARDROBE

• **Day skirt**: A solid 45" or 54" square of solid or print cotton. You can adjust length by folding *before* tying. Sarong-wrap at waist. For safety, secure it by adding a belt: a narrow canvas one, another scarf twisted and short-knotted, a length of hemp rope, etc.

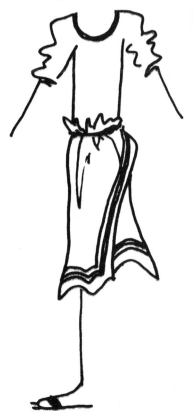

Wear with a T-shirt or blouse, i.e., white T-shirt, white-and-blue-cotton sarong skirt, red sandals — great-looking for *lunch on a boat or at a beach restaurant, or, just for an afternoon's shopping*, a blue cotton shirt, blue cotton print sarong skirt with straw bag and sandals are perfect!

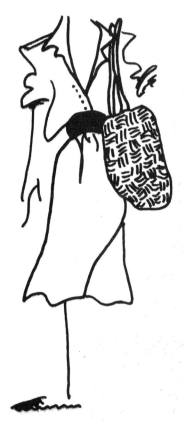

• **Evening: Bare Dress**: A flowered silk sarong skirt over *bare* black silk camisole belted in gold. Add gold sandals, cuffs and earrings. Divine at a restaurant (sexy!).

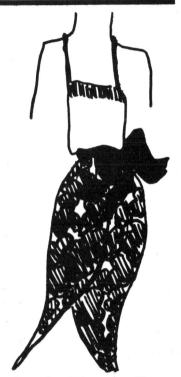

• **Scarf Dinner Dress**: Cream silk shirt, cream-wheat-and-tan-checked silk sarong belted in gold with gold sandals. Great warm weather night look for a dinner party at someone's home.

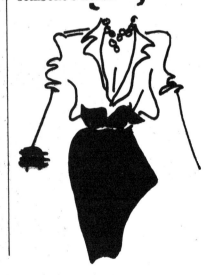

• **A Sarong:** Fabulous and sexy beach look: Take a large (45″ or 54″) cotton square, fold it on the diagonal, and hip-tie over a bathing suit. (Wear it also with only a T-shirt, sandals, and bikini bottom underneath. You'll find the result is an alluring look for beach lunches.

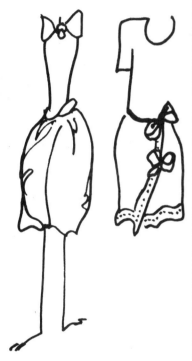

• **Summer Ways with Scarves:** Wear big extra-long cotton scarves (the 54″–60″ wide variety) as beach covers, for breakfast in the morning as an alternative to a robe, or after a bath while doing your makeup! Wrap and knot at bosom. Wear a robe, beach skirt, beach dress over a bikini bottom!

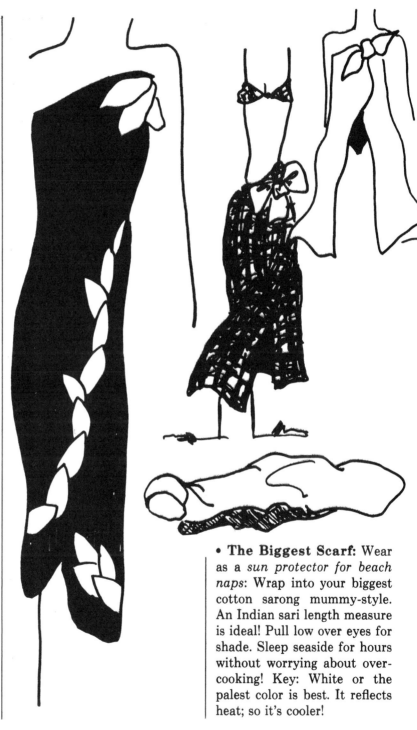

• **The Biggest Scarf:** Wear as a *sun protector for beach naps*: Wrap into your biggest cotton sarong mummy-style. An Indian sari length measure is ideal! Pull low over eyes for shade. Sleep seaside for hours without worrying about over-cooking! Key: White or the palest color is best. It reflects heat; so it's cooler!

123

BASIC SCARF WARDROBE

• Slide-knot a 45" or 54" silk square as a sarong over a silk shirt and narrow trousers, preferably matching . . . very Indonesian! *Fabulous for at-home dinners!* Try tan silk shirt and pants, violet-and-cream sarong, gold belt, jewelry, and sandals! *Or do it all white*: White silk shirt and pants with cream-and-white silk square as a sarong! Or all-black: black shirt and pants with a silk square of black-magenta-and-gold for sophisticated winter city at-home!

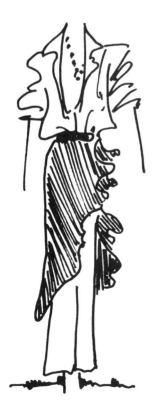

• *Summer "easy" version*: thin cotton 54" square striped narrowly in multi colors on white over white cotton T-shirt and thin white cotton drawstring pants. Add flat straw sandals and pretty bracelets. Nice way to look for *end-of-day drinks!*

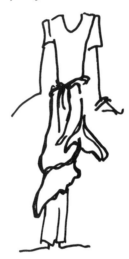

• *Tie a sarong at the waist over a dress* to change the look for daytime, when it's hot, and nighttime anytime! Key: Sarong must tone or match perfectly and must be thin, silky and airy! It is a second layer.

• Tie a navy and crimson cotton sarong over a navy cotton-knit bare dress for hot weather, add: bare sandals to go to *lunch in a hot place, a movie on a summer evening*, or to feel comfortable anywhere!

• Tie a sarong *over a silky bare look for evening*: Taupe silk strapless chemise-shaped dress, waist-bloused and tied with a dark rose-and-cream-georgette or thin silk sarong. Add gold belt and sandals! It is *a fabulous look for important drinks, chic dinners, etc.*

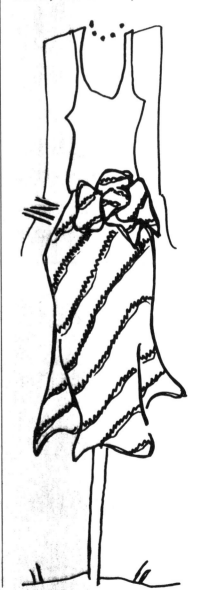

• Tie a sarong at bosom over narrow silk trousers, belt at waist, add gold for a *super dinner look* in resort, summer city, etc.!

• Bosom-knot a 54″ square *and wear it* as a *bare strapless dress*! A red silk sarong with wide black border which you waist-tied with a narrow rope of black cotton, gold jewelry, and bare gold sandals— *creates a sensational resort look*. Slide on a black silk cardigan as a cover, waist-tie with a black satin ribbon, add high-heeled bare black sandals, and you have *a perfect city restaurant look*! **Trick:** In case you just feel too undressed, simply slide a beautiful half slip underneath; match or tone it like an underskirt!

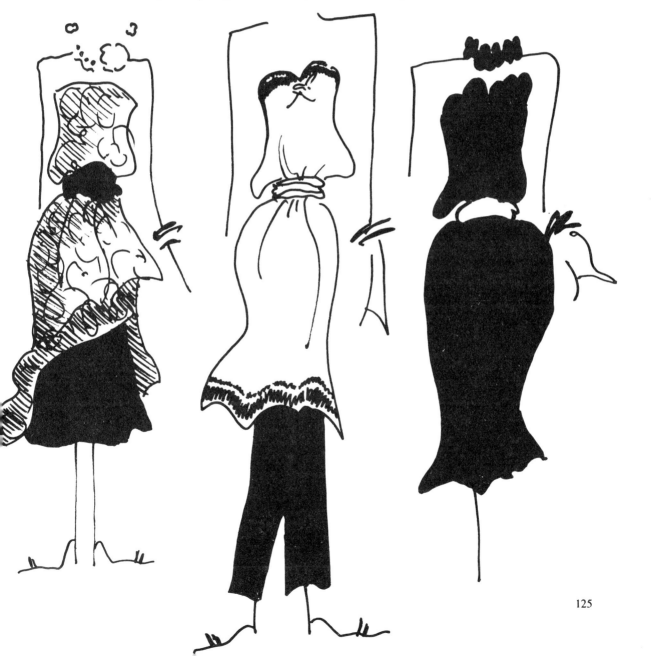

BASIC SCARF WARDROBE

• *Use silk and cotton scarves as evening covers!* Fold a 45″ or better, 54″—more to wrap into—on the diagonal and wear over your barest looks for cool night walks, air conditioning, or just added dash! When you don't want to wrap into it, fling it over one shoulder! Wear your prettiest silk ones or gauzy, thin, floaty cotton one for nighttime.

• **Proportion Note:** These are wonderful figure-problem distracters! A big silk float-of-a-scarf-shawl toned to what you are wearing slices into the silhouette and distracts the eye! Make sure it falls below the derriere when wrapped, however.

• *As a day cover,* cotton 54″ squares are great for country and city coverings over bare cotton-knit dresses or even a linen trouser and jacket turn-out!

• *Trick*: If you can handle it, when it's too hot to wear your shawl, an alternative look can be achieved by tying it around your hips like a giant bias tie. The effect is both dramatic and stunningly elegant, but this takes practice and a *slim* long body!

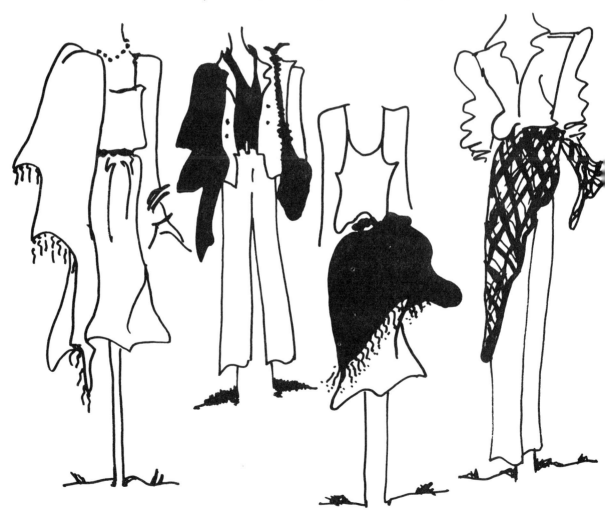

How To Wrap a "Sarong"

• *TIP*: Practice three or four times to get the feel!

• *Side-knotted* (easy with 54″ or 45″ squares) at bosom, at waist, or low on hips. Hold scarf behind you by both ends. Pull taut. Place sarong square where you want it. Bring top ends to meet, keeping tension as you pull ends together around body. Knot where you wish opening to fall: directly side, directly front, or off-center. Let the fabric fall loosely or waist-belt it if you are planning to wear at bosom.

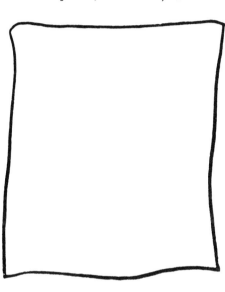 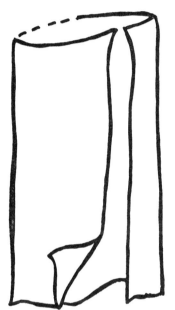 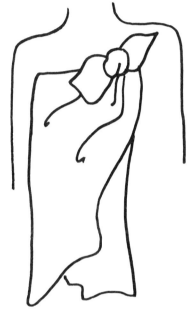

• *Side-wrapped* **in the Indonesian manner.** (1) Hold ends of sarong taut. Place where you want it—waist, hips, bosom. (2) With left hand, wrap sarong to right side, always maintaining tension in fabric with right hand. (3) Holding sarong in place at right side, bring fabric in right hand to center of body (or if you wish, a little off-center). Always maintain tension with both hands. (4) Gather up all the excess fabric with your right hand. Hold the excess at waist (or bosom if bosom-tying!). (5) Twist the excess fabric and, while tension is still held at *both* sides, tuck twisted end into waist or bosom.

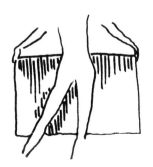 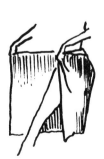 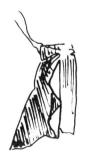 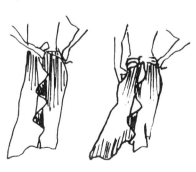

HAIR STYLE TRICKS

Quick Ways with Hair

• **Trick with bangs:** Sometimes they're fun, sometimes they're in the way. Have them cut long enough to reach mid-eyebrows and *not too thick*. This way you can flip them out of the way when you like—back off the face or combed to one side, etc. *For unruly bangs,* comb back off face with a comb dipped in diluted setting lotion (half water). Allow to dry. Brush tightly to smooth.

• INSTANT "LIFT" TO HAIR: Backbrush it over head all around. Flip hair back. Smooth down.

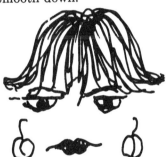

• **Instant Evening Hair:** Flip bangs into a slight winging curl with a curling iron. Smooth rest of hair back behind ears or into a low nape of neck tail. Tie with a black satin bow or bow tie made of narrow gold cord. Wear *pretty* earrings, *divine* evening make-up!

More Instant Evening

• Slick hair back off face. Tie

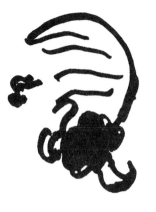

it with satin ribbon bow. Tuck a flower in bow.

Or fold and twist hair into a knot at nape of neck. Stick in some pretty hairpins to hold knot. Hold flyaway sides flat with pretty haircombs (gold, lacquered-colored ones, etc.).

TRICK *when wearing hair up or back:* To smooth down ends at hairline, sides, nape of neck, dampen a bit of cotton with diluted hairspray and touch lightly over hair . . . or slick lightly with fingertips just "touched" with pommade. It makes hair look nicely glossy too!

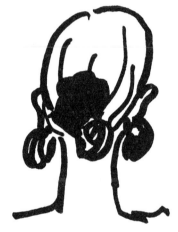

• **For more radical "sleek,"** comb hair through (back off face) with a comb dipped lightly in setting lotion. Smooth into slick shape: a chignon, a small nape-of-neck "tail." Allow to dry. Tuck a flower into the chignon knot or the rubberband holding tail . . . a camellia, gardenia, tiny white or pale pink orchid, a pale mauve "sterling silver" rose.

TRICK: for easy chignon knot, especially if you haven't long hair—a fine transparent hairnet! Tie hair back with rubberband. Attach net to top of rubberband. Then twist net and tail together into a knot. Wind excess net behind knot. Secure with more hairpins. It works!

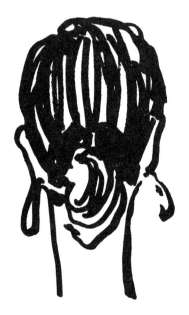

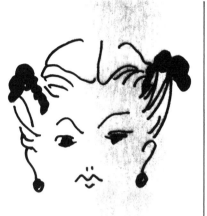

• Remember **Scarves!** Think of a luxurious gold one or dark, jewel-colored silk one for night. Pull hair back into tail. Twist scarf into long, tight snake. Tie as you would a ribbon around head. Knot at top center of head. Twist and bow-tie at nape of neck. Do a day version with a pretty paisely or a striped scarf!

Evening

• Smooth hair behind ear. Try a surface slick with fingers lightly touched with pommade just to give hair control and a hint of shine! Hold back with a pretty clip or comb.

• Day hair: Hold sides smooth with tortoise-shell-colored combs.
• *Classic day head:* loose, smooth, sleek shiny hair held off face with a black satin ribbon—very Chanel! *For evening:* tuck a tiny white camellia or small opened rose in knot of bow!

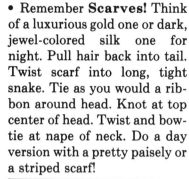

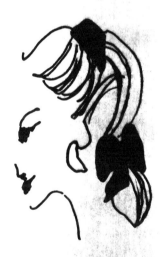

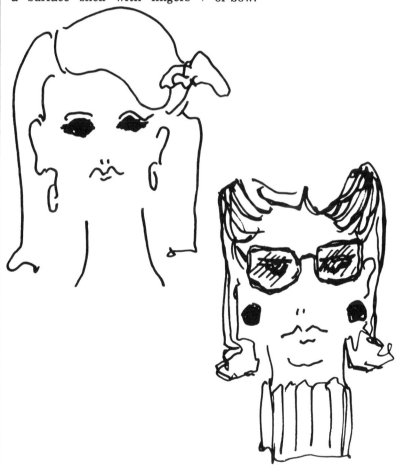

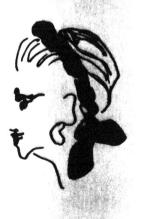

HAIR STYLE TRICKS

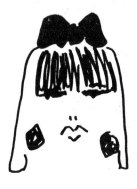

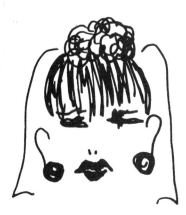

QUICK TRICK: Try pulling hair back into a knot while still wet—*great summer after-beach-shower hairdo.* Allow to dry to shape. Hold with a flower, pretty combs, hairpins, etc.

Setting TRICK: *for blunt straight hair:* While wet, lift sides and hold in place with combs. When dry release combs, brush up and out. The result is a nice "lift" to sides without a whole hairset routine!

Note: With all these quick tricks, perfect makeup and pretty jewelry (especially earrings) are vital!

To Collect for Instant Hair Looks

• **Combs in pairs:** gold, silver, lacquered ones in colors—scarlet, black wrapped with gold thread, violet, wine, pale ivory, shell colors of barely pink, and creamy apricot for summer! Tortoise plastic, carved bone, *real ivory* if you can find it! Black jet dotted with rhinestones for evening!

• **Narrow headbands of** colors and tortoise plastic. Ribbon-covered headbands: black satin, scarlet grosgrain, brown grosgrain, etc.

• Have a "wardrobe" of lengths of ribbon: longer ones to tie around head, short lengths to tie around nape-of-neck "tails" and bow á la George Washington. For fat bows: ½" wide, 1" wide, 1½" wide. Black satin, black grosgrain, brown satin, wine satin, navy satin, dark magenta satin . . . bright turquoise and scarlet ribbon!

• Use cording to tie around head and to wrap and tie around "tails" . . . narrow satin cording—black, gold, red, etc. . . . leather cording—tan, cream colored, brown, etc. . . . metallic cording—gold and silver!

• **Hairpins** (especially if you make chignon knots!): tortoise plastic, scarlet lacquer, wood—all colors and tones of wood!

• **Barettes**—gold, colors of plastic, bone, tortoise, etc.—to lift and hold sides of hair or to clip over short ponytails, etc.

• **Covered rubber bands!** Never use the regular stationery store rubber bands in hair. They are torture. They cut, break, and tear hair!

• **Beautiful fake flowers** if you can find them: A small silk gardenia, or a camellia. They can be very handy on a last-minute "whip - yourself - together-fabulously" hairdo!

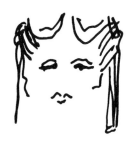

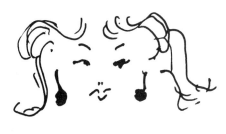

BELTS

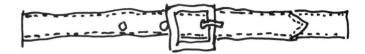

• **Important:** *For belts to work best they must relate in tone to your basic shoe wardrobe, day/evening!*

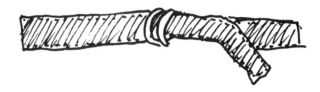

Pigskin or caramel leather/ brass buckle: to wear with trousers, jeans, skirts, country looks.

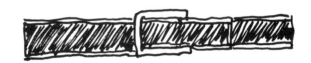

Brown soft kid belt (dressier day): for trousers (especially when you belt an overtop), skirts, dresses. For more mileage, select ones with matching leather-covered buckles. Then you can wear them with any jewelry (gold, silver, etc.) without risk of a clash of metal colors.

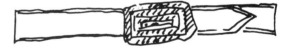

Black-edged with gold is indispensable for *evening*.

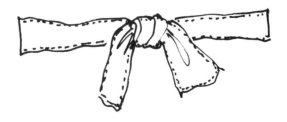

Gold kid or bronze, if your evening shoe is bronze! Or silver, if you've silver shoes. Add scarlet or emerald. Cobalt kid for a slash of color, depending on your other evening sandal colors!

BELTS

For Summer Add:

Natural-colored cotton canvas edged in leather (for trousers, jeans, summer country dressing).

A pale tone of leather **toned to day sandal color.**

A belt of rope, braided hemp, or straw to wear with cotton city looks and summer beach or country clothes!

White, or red, or bright blue kid (*depending on sandal colors*) for a **slash of color,** summer day and evening.

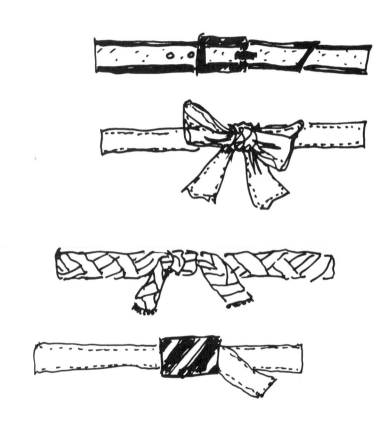

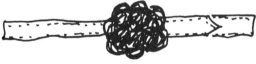

Tips—Belts

• **Make sure *basic belt wardrobe* relates *carefully* to *basic shoe wardrobe*!** If you own a red kid sandal, find a red kid belt. There will be the time when the two *together* will work a change of look—perfectly and effortlessly. To have on hand always: a gold belt for gold sandals, bronze for bronze, etc., for the same reason! Of course, you can use them separately too—brown shoes, a bordeaux belt, or gold sandals and black suede belt. That depends on what jewelry and colors you are wearing as well as your body proportions.

• *Keep belts on the narrow side for long life (and* narrowest for wide waist/hip problems! 1″–1½″ is perfect for day belts—the pigskin with brass buckle kind or ones that are leather with covered buckles. Ideal size for soft kid ones is between 1–¾″–2–½″ as they usually crush down when you put them on correctly.

• If you have waist/hip problems, 1/2″–3/4″ wide is best and *always toned* to what you are wearing! Your shoe can then be the slash of color *alone*

132

if you want it!

• If you *do* have a wide waist/hips and crave a *touch* of gold, try the **narrowest shoe-string of** gold kid tied loosely at the waist—never tight or you will look like a pillow tied in the middle!

• **For maximum mileage,** chose belts with matching covered buckles. You tire of them less, and they are more flexible for accessory changes.

• **Guidelines:** Start with a belt the *width of waistband. If you are short-waisted* and want torso length, *match* your belt to the color or tone of your top. Wear it a fraction on the loose side so that it sits low—just skimming below your natural waist. Be sure your waistband does the same; you don't want it to show above the belt!

• *If you are long-waisted* do the reverse: *Match* your belt to the color or tone of what you are wearing on the bottom (skirt or trousers).

TRICK: For the *illusion of a narrower waist*, put on the narrowest strip-of-a-belt, toned to what you are wearing, with a *pretty* buckle (day or evening!). The buckle draws attention to midwaist and draws the eye away from sides.

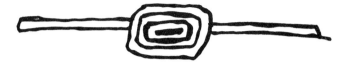

• **For day:** a brass or gold buckle on a toned kid shoestring belt.

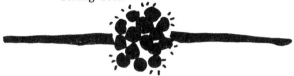

• **For evening:** a glittery buckle or one of colored stones on black suede if you wear black!

• **For summer:** a wood or woven straw buckle on hemp rope.

TRICK: you can do the buckle yourself with a favorite pin or clip. If the belt is narrow and supple, slip a pin over the front closing! If it ties at the waist, so much the better. Pin your pin into the knot or knot the belt at the back of your waist, especially if you are wearing a jacket to hide the knot, and pin the pin in front!

• *If you are short or short-waisted, remember to always tone belt to what you are wearing.* Always remember not to clip on anything too massive!

• **Trick for summer or warm places:** Tie the waist of a cotton T-shirt dress or solid silk dress with **a pretty scarf.** Wear the scarf point at your back and short knot the scarf in front. The best size: find the right size scarf to wrap your waist and end in a *short knot*; this way you have no rabbit-ear hanging ends! Depending on your size, proportions, and preference you could use flowered cotton, striped cotton, or *bright* solids! White cotton squares that are just piped with color along the edges are fresh and pretty. They can look smashing with a

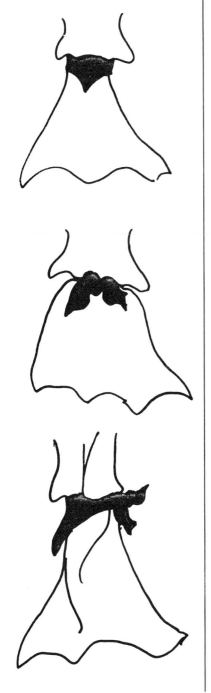

white T-shirt and white cotton skirt! *If you are narrow-waisted and narrow-hipped* this is a good look to try with a *one-piece maillot bathing suit!* **Do silk versions for evening,** or fold and twist a cotton or silk scarf and run through the belt loops of a skirt or trousers. Short knot the scarf in front. *For evening* try pinning a pretty pin or flower to the knot!

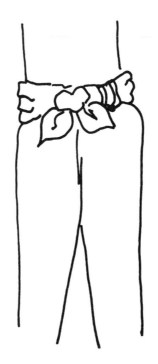

• *Pretty instant-evening look:* **To "turn" day into evening when you are wearing sweater and pants, run a long** *bias* **"muffler" of** *chiffon* **or silk through beltloops.** Magenta silk with black pants and black sweater. Do this *only* if you can stand the cut of color at the waist! Or wear a scarf of pale peach silk with gray flannels and a gray sweater.... Tie it in a bow at the waist. The "bias" insures the extra-pretty soft fall of a bow. *For more charm,* tuck a fresh flower in the knot...a camellia, baby orchid, nearly full-blown rose!

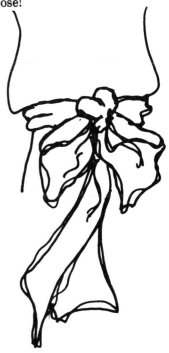

Trick: Instant Summer Day Belt—a rope! Buy a length in any hardware store: white cotton rope, package-wrapping hemp, even clothesline if it's soft and pliable enough! Knot the raw ends. It's a great way to waist-tie jeans, cotton T-shirt dresses, etc.!

• **Evening Version of the Rope:** Buy narrow rayon or satin cording. They come in amazing colors off spools in ribbon stores! Knot the ends. Wear **several** in one color or mix colors ... three tones of

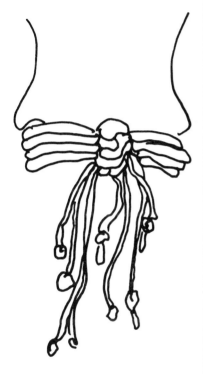

peach with pale gray silk ... red and orange with navy cotton. Make sure ends don't hang too long. No more than 6" from waist-knot to end-knot is about right. Or bow-knot all the lengths together at your waist!

• **More "Rope":** Bow-tie a length of leather or suede cording at the waist. It looks fabulous with a cotton T-shirt

dress or silk shirtdress! You can buy cording off spools in ribbon or jewelry supply stores. Note: All these "rope tricks" are great for wide-waist problems because the ropes and cordings are so narrow!

• **Do the same with *ribbon*: *Real* silk, double-faced is key! *It must look luxurious* and it will tie most beautifully—never look raggy!** Try black silk satin ribbon or colors of satin ... bordeaux to wear with black silk, pale gray to wear with cream or beige, pale peach to make gray flannel trousers look romantic. **Widths:** from 2"–3" or 4" wide in belt. Remember, when you tie the ribbon, it tends to crush a little. Waist-wrap the ribbon and tie it in a perfect bow—not too big, not too skimpy! *Trim the ends after* you tie bow! This way you can control the perfect length and bow size. A satin ribbon bowed at the waist can be the perfect finish for something as "big-time" as a bare black chiffon evening dress. (The best designers often do just exactly

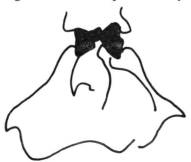

this to belt their prettiest evening looks!) Wrap a thin black velvet jacket closed with a dark wine satin ribbon. Waist-tie a printed silk shirtdress in pale rose tones with a ribbon of taupe rose satin!

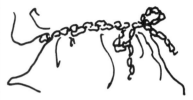

• **For more charm** tuck a flower in the bow-knot. A black dress or black silk trousers and sweater, waist bow-tied in black satin ribbon, and a white gardenia or pale pink camellia tucked in the knot of the ribbon are fabulous!

TYING TRICKS: How to tie scarves: Twist scarves *before* waist-tying. This helps "hold" the waist more neatly, and puts smaller amount of fabric spanning the waist, avoids a thick, "bunchy" look at sides. Do this twist with oblong scarves as well as squares.

• *Always fold square scarves along the bias* (diagonally) of the square *before* waist-tying. You want the fabric to be as narrow as possible, to pull through belt loops, for instance. First fold the opposite ends of the square in towards the center. Then do the diagonal-bias fold. Twist scarf and then waist-tie it.

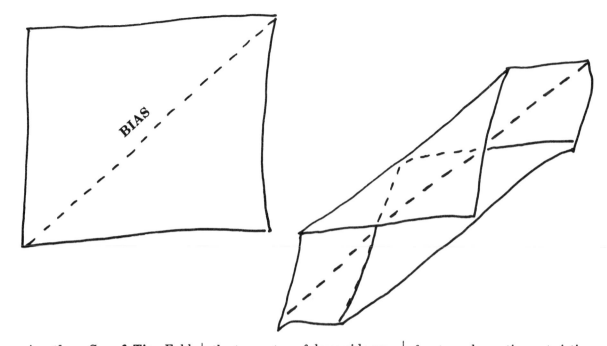

BIAS

• **Another Scarf Tie**: Fold square as above. Twist and wrap it around your waist while holding the scarf taut so that it remains as neat and narrow and "unbunchy" as possible. Knot at center front of waist. *Tuck loose ends in.* This is particularly important to do with a larger square. **Remember to twist ends before** you tuck them for a neater, tighter hold! Practice this one, however. The scarf "rope" should twist closely and evenly and the ends should be hidden away to look right.

TIP: If you want to blouse a top or dress over a belt or waist-sash: (1) Before belting or sashing, lift your shoulders as high as possible. This makes the top or top of dress ride up. (2) While your shoulders are lifted, belt. You then have an even excess of fabric above the belt. (3) When you relax your shoulders, you should have the perfect bloused amount. **Careful:** Be sure to check that the hem of your top or dress is even all around and that gathering is evenly distributed. Always gather a little more toward center front, the least but balanced amount at sides and back for *maximum slimness!*

• **Belt Trick:** Try twisting together two **(or several) colors of *flat* cotton or rayon cording or braid** (found in ribbon/dressmaking supply shops). Knot them in front and continue twisting the ends while you tuck them out of sight under belt! For evening try *two* or three tones of a color: taupe and cocoa or rose and pink. This can make the easiest, quickest, and most charming "finishing touch" to your turnout.

NOTE: With any of these Waist-tie "Inventions"— scarves or cording or ribbon— remember: they must hug the sides of the waist neatly, never look thick or bunchy. *Remember the number one trick:* Hold them taut by each end as you wrap and tie to help achieve smoothness. The key to the eventual ease of handling them is *practice.*

SHOES

Day—City
Winter

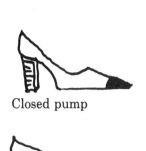

Closed pump

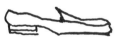

Trouser shoe (or low boot)

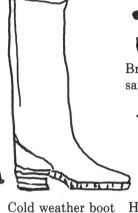

Rubber boot

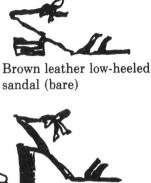

Cold weather boot

Summer

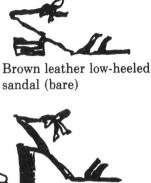

Brown leather low-heeled sandal (bare)

High-heeled sandal (brown- peanut leather)

Day—Country
Winter

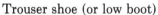

Flat moccasin (for skirt/pants dressing)

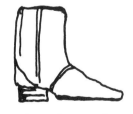

Short jeans/trouser boot

Summer

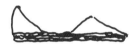

Espadrille (canvas and rope-soled)

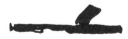

Flat sandal (pale beige leather)

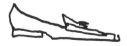

Moccasin (*pale* beige)

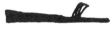

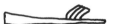

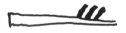

Add: Red kid, white, and gold kid sandals

SHOES

Evening—City

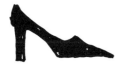

High-heeled black satin pump

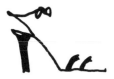

High-heeled black satin sandal

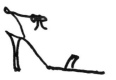

Bare gold or bronze-kid sandal

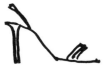

Add: Red or emerald satin bare high-heeled sandal or pump with heel

Evening— Country

High-heeled gold-kid or bronze sandal

Gold-kid or bronze flat sandal (also for day-summer)

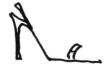

Add: Red or emerald-kid high-heeled sandal

over your stockings. Rubber does not "breathe." The socks help absorb perspiration!

• **Remember:** You don't have to *match* shoes to what you are wearing; you do want to *tone* them! The big help here is *a stocking toned to shoe color.* For example: a bordeaux-colored skirt, cocoa-colored shoe and stocking; a black skirt, brown-toned shoe and stocking. If you wear a black shoe with a black skirt or dress, **always** wear a stocking with a *tint* of black! The contrast between the black skirt, your skin tone (unless you are dark-skinned!) and black foot is too strong!

• *When not to tone a stocking to shoe?* when you are wearing a bright-colored shoe—too much color! When you are wearing white shoes (unless you are a nurse), always wear a skin-toned stocking!

• **The Best Neutral Day Colors:** tan, luggage-brown, peanut, dark cocoa... They will work with most day tones from black to gray to navy to dark wine.

TRICK: *Tone bag and/or belt to shoe.* This way you tie everything together!

• **Best Neutral Evening Colors:** metallic gold, bronze, dark steel.

• **The Neutral Summer Colors:** pale beige, tan, light luggage.

• *For longest legs:* A skin-toned color. A *tint* of color, peach, celery, mocha, etc., makes you look as if your leg goes on and on. Remember, white can be as stark as black—it attracts the eye to your foot! Wear white only if you are long-legged! Besides, a *tint of color* is more fun! *Remember: one long unbroken line!*

Your stocking should be the color of your shoe when the shoe color goes darker than your skin tone to keep the contrast from leg to shoe from being abrupt—one long unbroken line!

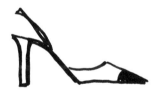

• ***The most elongating shoe shape:*** sling-back with a pretty, not-too-high, curved "throat," a nicely tapered toe, a *slim* medium high heel. *Too high a heel makes calf muscle too prominent so that short legs look shorter, as if you are on stilts, and heavy legs look heavier!*

• *For leg length:* Aviod T-straps, wide instep straps on sandals. Remember, ankle straps cut the leg in the worst place. If you can avoid them, the shoe (a sandal) and the strap must be as delicate as possible (a thread!), and the color must be close enough to skin color so that the shoe virtually disappears! A pump with a high throat or a shoe that laces up high is a leg shortener. Only wear them with trousers and socks to match color of shoes. Avoid anything heavy that breaks the line of flow from leg to toe. ***The goal: light, slender, and as delicate as possible—one long unbroken line!***

• *For illusion of length:* The ideal moccasin is one with a *bit* of a heel, even for the country. It makes your legs look better!

• *Avoid:* Low-throat shoes with trousers, especially for day. If you can't avoid, always *match* your stocking or sock to shoe color to avoid the flash of skin at ankle and instep! (Think of the look of a boot!)

• *For longest leg, avoid:* High-throated and lace-up shoes with skirts unless you have endlessly long legs, and then only if you *match* stocking *exactly* to shoe color. Otherwise they cut your leg and look too clunky! High-throated lace-up shoes are terrific as *trouser-shoes*—they give the line and look of a boot. Wear them with

SHOES

matching socks or stockings so that when you sit with your legs crossed you have a nice continuation of tone up your leg!

• *Avoid overly decorated shoes if you want leg length!* Bows, sparkle, etc., attract eye to shoe and instantly shorten the leg!

• *You Can Wear Low Heels If You Are Short If*: you make legs look as long as possible. *For skirts*, a *toned* stocking is a must. *For trouser dressing*, a lean-legged trouser or narrow jeans toned to shoe and stocking and *always* a top that is not overpowering! Remember: the bigger and bulkier the top, (coat, sweater, etc.), the more length you need or else you will look top-heavy!

• ***Do Not*** **wear dead-flat shoes if you have heavy legs!** Always think heel—even ½″ to 2″ helps.

• **For "big-time" dressing:** *never* dye shoes to match dress! It looks old-fashioned! If you want the *same color* family *do* dye shoes a *tone darker* so they don't look "married" to your dress. This, of course, does not apply to black or navy dressing! For pale chiffon or any "ice cream" color of silk, etc., a gold or silver sandal will look better than any ice-cream-colored shoe!

Tips on Shoe Care

Give new leather boots and shoes a slick of neutral cream polish or saddle-soap massage *before* you wear them—for protection! For soft kid leather, use cream polish; for stiffer saddle leather, saddle soap. Use a cotton flannel, not brushes, to buff. Polish shoes at least once a week or more after you wear them. This insures a long and attractive life!

Check boots and shoes regularly. *Do heel repairs, etc., before it's crucial!* Aside from looking terrible, a run-down heel will knock off the balance of shoe, put an *uneven* strain on it and contribute to wear! (Also will put a strain on your back!)

Brush suede boots and shoes with suede brush *after* each wearing. You can get these at your local shoe repair shop.

Trick for grease stains on suede: Shake a good amount of white talcum powder (or cornstarch or even *salt*, in a "pinch") on stain as quickly as possible after spattering. This helps absorb the excess grease. Allow powder to sit *without rubbing* for at least fifteen to twenty minutes. Shake off excess powder. With a stiff suede brush, brush the spot gently in a circular motion to start, then in one direction (against the nap), then in the other (with the nap). Sometimes the soft side of an emery board can help with very bad stains. Rub gently in a circular motion. The emery board actually scrapes the stained nap away, so be sure to **be gentle** and do only a little at a time!

Stuff wet boots and shoes with tissue paper or newspaper (absorbent!) and dry away from direct heat and light—never near radiators or open fires! This dries out the leather.

Store boots and shoes with proper boot and shoe trees (or soft paper stuffed in toes of shoes) to keep them from curling out of shape.

Stocking Tips

• *For maximum leg length always* tone stocking to shoe—with or without matching the skirt or trouser!

When wearing a dark shoe and skirt, *tone all three*—the stocking, shoe, and skirt—i.e., a black skirt and black shoe: black-toned leg always!

• When testing a stocking shade in a store, pull over the *inside* of your forearm. It is closer to leg color than the back of your hand. Like your legs, your forearm has less exposure to sun and weather. Look at the color in *natural light*, especially if you're buying tones for day. Take the stockings into the street if you must! Remember: Fluorescent light changes color values. This is important to know for any color decision! Fluorescent light has a blue cast. A color will look totally different in it than in natural day light, or in incandescent light!

• The best leg color for stockings is one that makes your legs *look slightly tanned* unless you already are! Watch out for stockings that give off a yellow or orange cast—or a gray or whitish one if you are dark-skinned!

• When toning stocking to shoe, bring your shoe along to the store. It is hard to impossible to "remember" color, much less an exact tone!

TIP: When you find the right tone for you, buy a lot. It saves time searching for replacements to your perfect stocking color!

• Make sure you have a supply of *sandalfoot* stockings to wear with sandals day and evening. The *worst look* is a bare sandal with a full-fashioned stocking toe—*Never*! Some women buy *only* sandalfoot for everything

so that there are no last-minute surprises when you are in need of a pair of stockings and the only one left with a sandalfoot has a run!

• **Textured stockings:** If your legs are heavy or short, *avoid* heavy-looking stockings and socks. For slimmer legs and the illusion of length, *do* try to find *sheer*, finely vertical-ribbed stockings. Tone them to the color of your shoe! Vertical lines narrow the leg!

• Always keep stockings proportioned to shoe. Avoid heavy-textured stockings with delicately shaped shoes, i.e., refined pumps or sling-backs. They make your legs look extra heavy and are all wrong! Wear heavily textured stockings only with country slacks, trouser shoes, or boots.

TRICK: With thin, silky fabrics or jersey and *especially* anything bias or clingy, wear *seamless panty hose with an opaque* "panty." They eliminate the need for underwear; therefore, you have no underpinning lines! For an extra slim, smooth line, try to find panty hose with a "support panty."

• **Trick:** When wearing trousers or jeans, you will have an easier, less binding fit through seat, crotch, and upper legs *if* you wear an underpant that

goes from your waist to top-of-thigh (smoother line this way!) and knee-high stockings (or knee socks!) instead of wearing panty hose. Stick to panty hose, though, if you are wearing any thin, clingy trouser or pajama!

Tips on Stocking Care

Store stockings in nylon-mesh bags or cotton ones. You can sew them yourself with big cotton squares! THE POINT: It keeps them from snagging in drawers and is also a good way to organize them!

(1) Keep tones separate. (2) Keep patterns and socks separate.

If you machine-wash stockings, wash them in a nylon-mesh bag (no snags!) If you hand-wash, watch out for rough spots around sink drains. Remove finger rings, etc. This too reduces the chance for snags!

Always put your stockings on *before* you put on jewelry!

Make especially sure that your toenails are smooth, callouses pumiced *before* you put on stockings. Nothing is more frustrating than to walk out the door and notice one toe poking through your stocking!

HANDBAGS

City—Day Winter

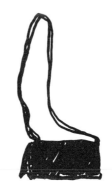

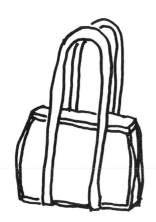

Shoulder bag—The tote/ "briefcase"—in a tone of brown or caramel-tan leather or tan canvas with brown-leather piping.

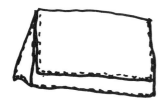

Envelope bag—soft kid—to carry inside shoulder tote in a tone of brown, caramel, etc., to go to lunch, etc.

City—Evening

Black satin or black silk small envelope.

Gold or bronze, depending on evening sandal metallic!

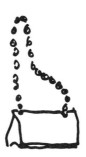

Add: Scarlet satin or whatever color matches your satin evening sandals.

Country—Day Winter

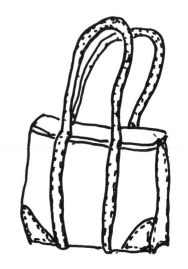

Dark caramel leather or canvas and leather.

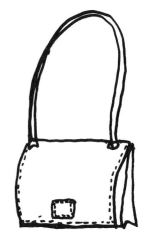

Dark caramel leather or pigskin.

Country—
Evening

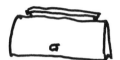

A brown tone of *soft* suede or kid envelope. Add an amusing color: Scarlet or Emerald kid!

Gold or your evening metallic sandal color.

Summer/Resort (City/Country)

Day

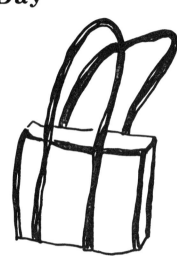

Pale cream or beige canvas-and-tan leather or all-canvas. Shoulder tote/briefcase.

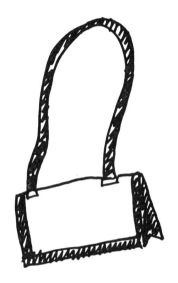

Canvas and leather or a tone of *pale peanut* to match day sandal.

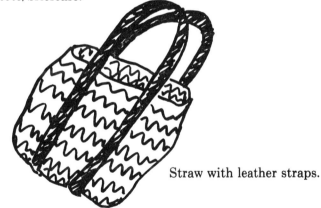

Straw with leather straps.

Evening

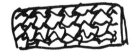

Small straw envelope.

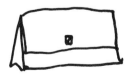

A pale color kid or scarlet kid small bag, depending on your evening shoe colors.

HANDBAGS

- In order for handbags to work well for you, *always tone or match them to day and evening shoes.*

- *Buy the best*! With proper care, leather improves with age. The better the quality, the longer it will last and the more beautiful it will become!

KEY: Test a bag before you buy it! Will it hold what you carry all day? Evening? Nothing is worse than the moment you are out the door and your compact and glasses won't fit in your evening bag! *Remember, a bag becomes a part of you.* You carry it *on* you—and you are constantly using it! Does it feel comfortable on your shoulder, under your arm? Can you *see* into it easily? (The old story of "where *are* those keys!") Can you comfortably organize "your life" in your handbag?

- *Evening trick*: Keep a complete set of evening bag essentials on hand, either in one evening bag which you use constantly or in *a small box, readily at hand* to fill any evening bag quickly ... a small comb, money—one $5 bill (for taxis), some dimes (for phone calls), quarters (for ladies room tips), a small compact of powder, lipgloss for touchups, an *extra set* of house and car keys on a tiny bit of ribbon (your *essential* keys only, to fit in any small evening bag). This trick saves the awful last-minute fumble and avoids the disaster of forgetting anything. *Be sure to test "essentials"* in all your evening bags to make sure they fit!

- **Handbag Organization Tip:** A *spare eyeglass case* makes a great holder for a small hairbrush and/or comb—keeps them clean and easy to get at, and prevents them from scratching leather items in your bag! It also makes a great holder for *pens and pencils*—keeps them within easy reach *and* avoids the disaster of felt-tip pen or ballpoint marks all over your wallet and the inside of your bag when pen tops accidentally come off!

- **Organize your wallet:** Keep big bills *separate* from small bills. You know what we mean if you've ever given a taxi driver a $10 bill thinking it was $1. A wallet with an outside change purse attached to it is ideal (rather than a separate change purse)—saves time and fumbling!

- **Ideal case for keys:** A key ring that slips into its own pouch—keeps keys from scratching everything in your bag.

- *Key trick for large-handbag users:* To find keys quickly, slip them onto their holder and then into a brightly colored extra eyeglass case. Or attach a bright-red cotton, fringed tassel—the kind you buy in upholstery shops to put on drawer keys or for hanging from drapery ties—to the end of your key chain. This way you will have a better chance of seeing them in the "dark depths of your bag!"

- If You Carry a Lot With You in a Day: Look for a handbag with gussets that expand. Make sure the bag is wide enough to carry your largest and widest daily item: a legal pad, your daily calendar, your newspaper, etc. Test it!

- If You Carry Your "Office" in Your Bag"—Some people need to: a tape recorder, calculator, camera, notebooks, agenda, depending on your job needs—Look for a *shoulder* bag:

- (1) which will hold all your needs easily, comfortably.

- (2) that is soft, lightweight, so that it doesn't add bulk and weight to what is already a "load."

- (3) that balances well on your shoulder when filled. *Test it!* This is the key to a successful bag purchase, especially since this kind of bag is expensive! Make sure the shoulder straps don't cut into your shoulder—Avoid overly narrow ones; they *do* cut! Make sure the straps don't slip off your shoulder when you are walking. This happens when bag does *not* balance when filled or when straps are too wide!

• (4) that holds, in *addition to your big work items, a smaller envelope bag*. In this you should keep your wallet, keys, glasses, beauty essentials (cosmetics in *their own little soft bag*), plus anything of value! It's safer . . . you know where everything is! *Note*: This smaller envelope is the bag you take to lunch. Leave the big carry-all bag in your office or *check it* at the restaurant so you don't feel as if you're carrying your suitcase to the table!

• *Ideal Day Bag Size*: To hold personal essentials, to go *inside* your big all-day carry-all: around 10″ × 12.″ *Remember, try it out no matter what*. It should hold all your essentials *without looking overstuffed*!

• *Trick Solution For a Working Bag*: A soft *pretty* leather briefcase to use as a handbag/tote. Some even come with a detachable shoulder strap! Or a soft leather zipper legal-size portfolio. These are designed to hold legal-size papers. The soft leather ones are more feminine for one thing. If they have an expandable gusset, they can hold in addition a small makeup case, an envelope clutch bag, eyeglass case, address book, daily calendar, etc. A classic, efficient and *good-looking* business-day solution!

• **Summer version of portable office-bag:** Look for hemp or woven-straw "shopping bags"—or those great-looking ones imported from Africa or the Far East, which cost practically nothing. Find them in straw and wicker shops, ethnic boutiques—Indian, Japanese, African, etc.!

These are very attractive, functional and *relatively inexpensive*. Make sure you choose something sturdy enough to take the weight of your daily needs. (They also double as great *weekend bags* for carrying clothes to the country, vegetables and general shopping *in* the country, taking to the beach!) *Equally summery and efficient*: a canvas tote like the classic canvas icebag found in boat-supply catalogues, L.L. Bean catalogs, etc.! Put a canvas or cotton-printed envelope bag inside, one of canvas piped in pale leather, or a makeup bag of flowered cotton! It's a pleasant and inexpensive way to make everything pretty!

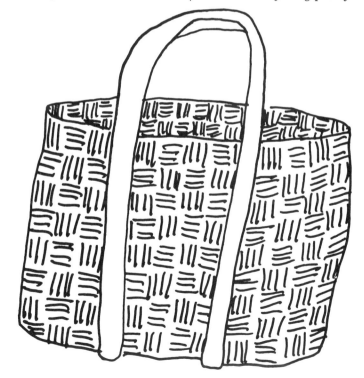

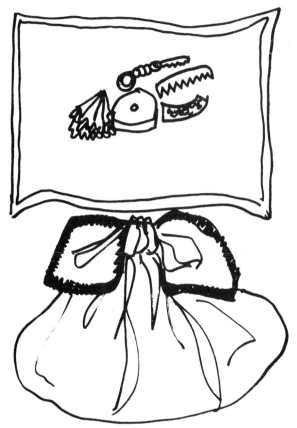

TRICK FOR INSTANT EVENING BAG: Put all your evening essentials in the center of a 10″ or 12″ square of silk or satin and tie it like a knapsack. First knot together end #1 and #2 then end #3 and #4. Make sure the fabric is not too thin or your "essentials" will poke through and look strange! If the fabric is thin, you can put two exact sizes together, one over the other, or buy a "weighty" piece of satin by the yard and have ends edge-stitched by machine. These squares are useful (and easy!) to have on hand for a last-minute DASH OF COLOR! In summer they could be squares of flowered cotton.... Chintz is ideal because of its weight and crisp "finish"!

Handbag Care

• As with boots and shoes, polish leather bags with a good neutral-colored cream leather polish and buff with a soft cotton flannel (not a brush!) *before* you use them! Don't forget leather wallets, eyeglass cases, little purses, etc. Re-polish at least once every week or two depending on use! The more you care for them, the longer they will last and look beautiful! See "shoe care tips" for cleaning suede.

• **Remember:** When storing handbags, keep all leather bags in soft cotton flannel bags—**not plastic**, it dries the skin! Stuff bags with tissue to help them maintain their shape. *Be careful of metal clasps*, etc., especially if bags are closely stacked one next to the other, back to back. You risk marking soft leather by the pressure of anything metal or hard against it—even when protected by a flannel case!

• *Try spraying straw bags with Scotchguard* or other fabric-protecting spray—a light, quick, even coating. Allow it to dry well before you carry the bag. This keeps them from getting dirty and also waterproofs them.

• *If leather bags do get wet*: As with shoes and boots, stuff them with tissue or newspaper and dry *away* from heat and light. Do not overstuff—they could stretch out of shape! If your leather bags get water-spots, don't despair. The nature of leather, especially *good* leather, is that spots have a tendency to fade or disappear after a time. This is why an initial coat of polish *before* using leather is so important: it helps seal the surface!

GLOVES

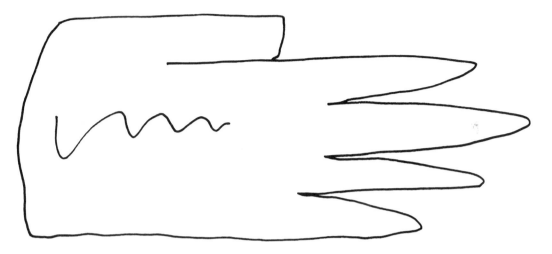

• *Classic Pigskin*: unlined, short to wristbone. To wear with trouser and skirt suits in the city; in the country with jeans and tweed blazer, suede jacket and wool skirt, etc.

• *Knit gloves*: cashmere, lambswool, etc.—Beautiful quality! They are nice if you can find mid-forearm length to crush down or cuff like a sweater. *To wear for warmth*!

• *Trick*: Buy knit gloves to *match* your basic sweater collection: black, beige, navy, red, ivory. They look wonderful matched to sweaters! Black and ivory can go beautifully formal at night!

• If you live or travel to cold places, have one pair of fur-lined or silk-lined leather or sheepskin gloves. To wear on zero-degree days and nights.

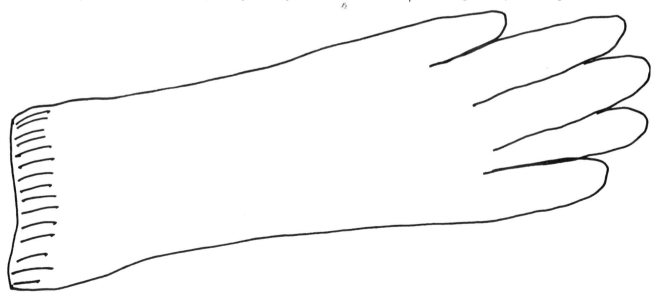

SKIN, HANDS AND –

Skin

A Simple Rule:
Good Skin Is the Basis of Good Makeup.

Basic Musts:

• **VITAL:** At night (*every* night!), remove makeup *thoroughly* . . . skin needs to breathe. **Spend time removing makeup carefully!**

• **VITAL:** Drink at least eight glasses of water daily!

TRICK: *After* cleansing and *before* moisturizing, hydrate skin with a fine spray of water (from a spray bottle). For a zipping morning lift and anytime you are in hot weather, keep bottle in refrigerator!

• *The best time to moisturize face and body is right after your bath.* Key spots to moisturize: eye area, around mouth, throat! *The way to moisturize:* Apply it, wait twenty minutes. Blot off excess. (For oily skin—5–10 minutes)

• SLEEP! Sleep with head elevated to keep skin under eyes from puffing. Try not to sleep with face on one side—makes wrinkles.

• **Remember:** Skin changes with weather, medicine intake, illness (fever), etc. You must adjust your skin routine with these changes in mind. Study

and "learn" your skin. *Use a magnifying mirror!*

• **VITAL:** A *well-balanced diet.* This is the key for everything from skin to hair to body function to mind function—vitamins, minerals, protein, etc.!

• **VITAL:** *Good circulation is for good skin tone.* How to get it? (1) Drink eight to ten glasses of water a day! (2) Masks, facials. (3) Brisk walking, jogging, exercise! (4) Body massage. *Avoid* vigorous massage or rubbing of facial skin—it breaks down musculature, can injure capillaries, etc. *Trick:* For a quick circulation stimulator, jog in place for one to two minutes *lifting legs high*, trying to touch chest with knees without leaning forward! Keep a steady breathing rhythm.

• Too much makeup blocks pores. **Keep a light hand.** For the sheerest amount, always apply foundation with a **water-damp silk sponge!**

Skin Recipes: TRICK: For *temperamental skin*: Steep two teabags. Wait until they cool to room temperature. Dab face with teabags for five min-

utes. Rinse off. Do three or four times a week.

• **Trick:** *For dry, itchy skin:* (overly air-conditioned or steam-heated atmosphere!) Wash face with superfatted soap. **Dab skin with milk.** Leave on five minutes. Rinse off. Or—try **oatmeal-and-water compresses!**

• *For sensitive skin:* Soak *cucumber slices in milk* for half hour. Remove from milk. Place slices all over face. Leave on twenty minutes. Rinse with cool water.

• *Oily skin*: (1) anti-bacterial soap, (2) astringent, (3) always oil-free *water-based foundation!* Use masks regularly. Clay masks are great; they literally absorb oil!

• **TRICK:** Petroleum jelly for **"crash moisturizing"** of extra dry spots—around eyes, mouth, neck, knees, elbows. Apply warm. Leave on one hour. **Do not remove!** Directly take a warm bath and soak five minutes to allow maximum penetration of moisturizer before soaping down!

• **Skin stimulator:** one teaspoon of thyme, one cup of

FEET

boiling water. Steep for ten minutes. Apply with cotton compresses to clean face. Leave on for 3–5 minutes. (Great just before doing evening makeup.)

• For dry skin spots, apply eye cream; cream elbows, knees, neck—then shower!

Body Moisturizing Tip

• **For dry or winter-dry body skin,** *avoid* soaking in hot baths. Take warm showers or quick warm baths only.

TRICK: Moisturize all over body **before** getting in bath. (Baby oil all is great!) Sit in warm bath for 2–3 minutes before soaping off. Reapply moisturizer while *body is still damp!*

Recipes for Beautiful Skin

• *Grated raw potato* eye compresses: Helps reduce eye swelling and dark circles. Relax—elevate feet!

• Cotton compresses soaked in *milk:* good tired-eye relaxer!

• *Tomato slices*: directly on skin for breakouts. Leave on for ten minutes.

• A mask of thin slices of *ripe bananas* over face for dry sensitive skin. Leave on ten minutes. Relax with feet **elevated.**

• **Avocado Mask:** Mash avocado all over face **if skin is dry.** Apply avocado to sides of face only. Use mask of **shredded apple** for oily "T" zone! (Forehead, nose and chin).

• **Cool camomile tea is the gentlest skin hydrator.** Steep some and keep a spray bottle of it in refrigerator. **Trick for removing masks:** Use room temperature camomile tea instead of plain water!

• Great oily skin mask: a paste of oatmeal, a squeeze of one-half a lemon, some mint leaves all blended together. Gently massage into oily places. Leave on 3–5 minutes. Remove with compresses of witch hazel or camomile tea.

Basic Skin Routine

Remember: "Routine" means regular, habitually! In order for skin to benefit from proper care, the routine must be followed regularly! Key: A gentle hand! Dab, touch lightly—never pull or rub skin, no matter what the step!

• A.M.
Clean skin with mild skin cleanser and cotton pads.

• Wash off residue with mild soap and *cool* water. Hot water is too hard on skin! *Dab dry.* Do not rub!

• Use tonic (or astringent if oily skin) to close pores.

• Apply light moisturizer (to neck, too!) **while skin is still damp.** It protects and hydrates skin and allows makeup to go on more easily. **Tip:** Allow skin to "settle" for 5–10 minutes before makeup. Begin dressing, etc.

• Do makeup.

P.M.
• Cleanse skin with cleanser and cotton pads. (Do not forget neck and eyes!)

• Wash off residue with **mild** soap and water.

• Apply a *richer moisturizer/ night cream* to dry parts of face: hairline, sides of cheeks, temples, neck.

• Apply (gently dab!) *eye cream* around eye area—lids and corners of eyes, under eyes especially.

• Apply a *light moisturizer* to T-zone (forehead, chin, nose). *If you have oily skin,* you might leave this step out!

• Leave creams on for a *maximum of twenty minutes.* Pat off excess cream. Leave on lids and eye corners, but remove **extra gently** from *under* eye area!

SKIN, HANDS AND FEET

Once a week: Use a mask. The best time is at night. You can leave skin free to breathe afterwards, instead of putting on makeup! Also, a home atmosphere is more pollutant-free, better for freshly cleaned skin!

Masks: **Note:** Masks are most effective if skin is gently steamed beforehand to open pores. Alternative to steaming: Apply mask **directly after a warm bath;** pores are opened from the warmth of the bath!

How to Steam

• Take a large bowl (or basin) of boiling water into which camomile or special facial steaming herbs have been added. (These can easily found in health food stores and good pharmacies!)

• Make sure face is clean.

• **Key:** Make sure a thin film of moisturizer has been dabbed on skin (especially eye area—lids!) for *protection!*

• Place a large towel over head and bowl to make a tent. Lean face over steaming bowl—never closer than 12" to the water. *Make sure steam's not too hot*—you should never feel a burning sensation. If you do *it's* too hot, lift towel/tent, allow steam to cool. *Make sure eyes are sufficiently protected*, as eye skin is extra-sensitive!

• Steam 3–5 minutes.

• Gently pat off moisture and moisturizer with tissues.

• Apply mask immediately.

About Masks

Moisturizing Masks
They do not dry on face. They cleanse, smooth, and help *moisturize* skin. Good for normal to dry skin.

Peeling Masks
They go on creamy and come off in one continuous sheet. Peeling masks are effective for skin smoothing, but most effective if skin is gently steamed beforehand to open pores. They remove dead skin cells, help clean out pores. Good for oily to normal skin.

Exfoliating Masks
These go on creamy. They are removed by gently rubbing in circular motion. *It is important to know in which direction to rub in different areas of the face:* (1) Up and out towards hairline, cheeks, temples, forehead. (2) Center and out towards sides, chin, sides of nose. (3) Up towards forehead and hairline, top of nose and center forehead. (4) Up and out, cheeks. (5) Up towards chin, throat. **Important:** Remove in **small bits** with small, gentle circles. No big pulling movements! Exfoliating masks cleanse dirt and dead surface cells. Excellent for oily *or* normal skin.

Drying Masks
These actually contain clay or silicas and dry hard on skin. They blot up oil, dirt, toxins. Remove with warm compresses of water or camomile tea. Great for *oily skin*. Use a mild astringent such as witch hazel to completely close pores after removing if skin is very oily. If skin is normal to dry, after removing mask apply a *light* coat of *light* moisturizer to skin to balance any drying effects of mask!

Skin Protection Tips

• **Key:** *Avoid Sun Exposure* (summer and winter!). Sunscreens, sun blocks; makeup with sunscreens should be as habitual as brushing teeth! Don't forget neck, hands, chest.

• *When you are in sun places*: (1) Remember, water intensifies sun rays! (2) Avoid sunning between 10 A.M. and 2 P.M. when the sun is strongest (Disaster time!). (3) **Head/hair/skin protection:** a wide brimmed hat—straw or white cotton—or a white cotton scarf. (White reflects heat; cotton is porous!) (4) Protect eyes, eye areas! Apply sun block on lids and around eyes and wear protective sunglasses!

• **For Cold Places: Remember:** Cold weather tends to dry skin. Always moisturize well before going outside. Add eye cream, hand cream! Protect lips with rich, lubricating gloss, lipstick or lip cream. Steam heat dehydrates! Use humidifiers and pans of water on radiators to add moisture to atmosphere!

• Never use makeup without moisturizer layer first. It keeps makeup from clogging pores, protects skin.

Hands
To Know:

• *The best nail length*: on the short side—about a ¼″ from tip! Looks efficient and intelligent. Long claws are definitely not appealing.

• *The best nail shape*: straight sides, slightly rounded at corners. If you get a snag, you have room to smooth it off! Oval and pointed nails make fingers look fat. They break more easily. Too square a shape makes hands look heavy and broad!

• *The best nail color*: depends on skin tone, length and state of health of nails. The best, classic, most efficient day looks are clear nail gloss and white stick under nails or a clear neutral pale tone. Wear *flashy colors* only at night and with discretion, or on *toes*—looks great with sandals in the sun!

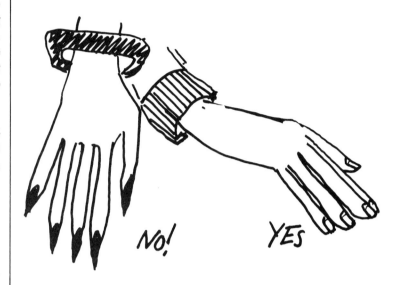

Nail Color Guide

Fair Skin: corals, soft pinks, pinky reds. *Very white pale skin*: avoid yellows (tawny colors). Stay with roses, pinks with blue undertones, pink reds, etc. *Olive (yellow-toned) skin*: amber, tawny apricot tones, true reds. *Dark olive skin*: Berry colors. *Black skin*: Warm raisin and berry tones (sharp screaming colors, no!).

Nail Protection Tips

• Never file nails after a shower, bath etc. They are too soft then. You risk splitting and peeling them.

• Use the *minimum* of nail polish remover. It's drying to nails, makes them brittle. Touch-up tips: Try using re-

mover only once a week for full manicure; moisturize nails well!

• Nail polish can help strengthen nails. It protects them. Remember, don't entirely remove polish—"touch up" when chips happen!

• Moisturize hands and nails and use cuticle creams as often as possible (twice a day minimum).

• Do a weekly warm petroleum jelly/white cotton gloves treatment. Sleep with it on!

• **For brittle nails,** try soaking them in warm olive oil.

• Use a sun screen on hands! Sun exposure to hands, like

sun exposure to face, is aging and dangerous!

• Never file nails into corners; it weakens them.

• Apply nail hardeners to tips only. This way you avoid possible allergic reactions!

• *If your nails are short, do not* **wear strong or bright-colored polish.** It only attracts the eye to stubby ends. Wear clear polish or a subtle skin tone . . . makes nails look longer.

• Protection: Use rubber gloves (cotton-lined to absorb moisture!) for washing dishes, all household chores, gardening. Or wear thin cotton gloves under unlined rubber gloves!

Trick: Apply a good slathering of hand cream and then put on rubber gloves. While you work you are giving hands a beauty treatment! Especially effective when washing dishes—the heat of the water helps cream to penetrate skin!

• *To clean discolored nails:* dip a cotton-tipped stick in lemon juice or hydrogen peroxide!

• **Protection:** Remember, wear gloves in cold weather—even if your hands aren't cold! Gloves keeps hands from getting dry and chapped.

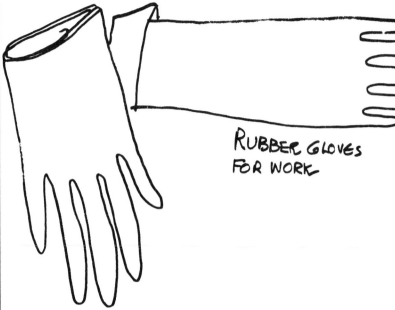

RUBBER GLOVES FOR WORK

WHITE COTTON FOR SLEEP

Feet

• **To Know:** After bath, dry feet well and powder. Never put on shoes and stockings with damp feet.

• Use a *pumice* every time you bathe or shower to **prevent** callouses and corns and rough spots from forming. Liberally coat pumice with moisturizer before using and several times during use. This keeps skin moist and helps slough off dry areas.

• "Preventive Medicine:" Watch for foot danger signs—blisters, red sore spots on toes, bottoms of feet. Are your shoes too tight? Don't wait; correct immediately *before* you have serious foot problems!

• Have *regular pedicures.*

• If your feet hurt: If you have serious bunions, callouses, etc., a foot doctor is the answer. There is nothing as debilitating as sore, sick feet. *Have them treated professionally.*

• *Overnight treatment* for extra dry, sandpaper feet: massage warm petroleum jelly into skin, wear white cotton socks.

• **Tip:** See shoe section for tips on **how** and **when** to buy shoes. Do Not Forget Feet: A pedicure is not a luxury, it's a *necessity,* especially if you are wearing sandals! It helps keep feet healthier. It's as important as having clean hair, skin, face and hands!

HAIR CUT/WASH/— PROTECT

The secret to great-looking hair:

1. Healthy hair and scalp. This means Perfect Condition!

2. A good cut.

Fact: There is no way to have pretty hair (style, cut, etc.) without first having *healthy* hair! *The basis of healthy hair/scalp*: vitamins, a balanced diet, exercise (for circulation)!

Note: Most hair salons today emphasize hair care—proper washing, conditioning, protecting—as much as hairstyle!

Hair Facts

To Know About:

• **Beware of city pollution.** City living means your hair needs regular *daily* washing and conditioning.

• **Beware of tension.** Scalp, neck, shoulder muscles tense and tighten. Blood flow is restricted. Oxygen supply is cut down. Hair/scalp immediately suffers. Professional massage of head and shoulder area helps. Learning the warning signs and learning to relax are vital!

• **Beware of sun!** Sun dries out hair. Avoid washing hair before going in the sun—natural oils help protect hair. Use a conditioner with sunscreen! Comb it through and leave it on. Slick hair back with combs or tie with a cord—chic!—or wear a hat or a cotton scarf turban. After sun, shampoo and *condition* always. Perspiration, salt water, and chlorine are terrible for hair!

• **Beware of cold weather.** Hair tends to dry out, like skin, from steam heat, too! It can become brittle from exposure to extremes of cold-to-warm-to-cold as you go outdoors, indoors, etc. Head coverings for cold protection keep air from getting to scalp. Hair/scalp must be treated and treated gently! Cold weather causes static electricity in hair. How to combat: Dampen brush before running through hair.

• **Beware of hair dryers.** Like strong sun and wind they damage hair. Always keep on medium to cool heat—not high!

• Hold at least one foot from hair. Keep it moving around rather than directing to one spot for too long a time. **Key:** Stop drying while hair is **slightly damp.** It's the time from damp to bone-dry when the real "burning" damage is done!

• **Beware of overbrushing.** Yes, forget one hundred strokes a night! Brush only to loosen hair (before washing for instance), to dress and smooth hair, or to backbrush (with head hanging down) a few strokes all around to give hair bounce. Use a brush with smooth bristles, never sharp, scratching ones! Same goes for combs. If the teeth are sharp they will only tear and damage hair! *Trick:* To remove dust and grime from city hair, pull an old nylon stocking over brush and brush back (head hanging forward) a few strokes in every section.

• **Remember,** scalp and hair can (and usually do!) have different characters. For example —oily scalp/dry hair. Or the reverse—oily hair/dry, flaking scalp. Have your hair/scalp analyzed by a professional, especially if you are having problems. This is the quickest way to finding the right recipe for you rather than hit-and-miss self-analysis and treatment!

• **Remember:** Hair, like skin, like fine china, should be treated gently. Never rub! Pat dry. Work shampoo in gently, never violent massage and rubbing! Comb gently. **Tip:** If hair tangles, comb hair from bottom up, working out tangles. Never yank!

HAIR CUT/WASH/PROTECT ———

- Dilute shampoo with water, especially if it's necessary that you wash your hair everyday. **Trick:** Decant into large plastic bottle. Dilute 50 per cent with water.
- If you wash your hair every day, shampoo only once.

- No matter what your hair quality—fine, oily, dry, bleached, etc. . . . *condition every time you wash*. There are conditioners formulated especially for different hair types/problems.

- **Do-it-yourself condition recipe:** one egg, equal amounts of castor oil and glycerine whipped together. Coat on hair. **How to apply conditioner:** Put conditioner on bottom two-thirds of hair—not scalp! Work in by separating strands of hair with fingers. Comb through with wide-tooth comb. Rinse out *well*. Trick: To completely remove traces of conditioner, add a little vinegar in next-to-last rinse, followed by a final *cool* rinse to "firm up" hair.
- Use cool to lukewarm water when washing hair—*never hot, never icy*.

- **Remember:** Stress, metabolic disorders, fever, hormone imbalance, nutrition imbalance, medicines, can affect hair and scalp problems. If you suspect any of these, see your doctor!

How to Wash Hair

A proper washing routine is key to healthy hair!
- Brush hair a few strokes to loosen grime. **Trick:** Brush in the direction you will wash—over head, from nape of neck forward if you are going to hang your head in a basin, or back from face if you're going to wash it in a shower with head back!

- Wet thoroughly with *warm*, never hot water!

- Apply diluted shampoo to hair. **Trick:** Pour shampoo into hands. Rub through hands first so that you apply shampoo evenly over head and not in one spot. Never *pour shampoo directly on hair*. You waste it.

- Gently massage shampoo through hair and scalp, making sure you work it through hair to ends. **Remember, hair is fragile!**

- Rinse thoroughly.

- Remove excess water from hair by throwing a towel over head and *squeezing* towel and hair gently. Never rub to dry.

- Apply conditioner to hair. Begin two inches from scalp and work it into hair—not scalp!—down to tips. Separate strands with your fingers to work it in

well. Comb through finally with a wide-tooth comb. Leave on whatever amount of time is designated for the conditioner.

- Rinse well. First with warm, *not hot*, water—then cool water. You may want to add a little vinegar to rinse just before final rinse-out to remove all traces of conditioner.

- Again—never rub hair to dry. Throw a towel over head and *gently squeeze*, or pat towel to remove excess water. Think of pure silk stockings! Gentle!

- To Untangle Wet Hair: Use a wide-tooth comb or brush with plastic rounded bristles in a rubber base. The bristles *bend* when they reach knot-resistance—they don't tear! *Gently* comb out hair. Trick: (1) Work from bottom tip of hair up. (2) Do head in sections: Begin at nape of neck, hold top hair up with one hand, and gently work out the underneath layers first.

Haircutting Guidelines

Secret #2 to great hair: *Great Haircut!*

The goal: Do-it-yourself hair—the kind for which you don't need to rely on a hairdresser to arrange "wonderfully." The kind of haircut that requires at most a few heated rollers to whip into shape in a pinch. Ideally the kind of haircut that you can wash, damp dry, flip around with your fingers or a brush, and go on your way . . . *that's modern hair!*

• A great cut makes thin hair look thicker, limp hair less limp, thick hair manageable.

• For thicker, stronger hair, a blunt cut is key, especially if you intend to wear your hair straight and smooth! This allows hair shafts to retain maximum moisture with less chance of split ends. Allows hair to swing in even line!

• **Tip: How to find a good hair cutter:** Whose hair do you admire? Ask *them* where they get their hair styled.

• **Tip:** The ideal haircutter wants to see his client *before* hair wash *while she's still dressed!* It's important to get the top-to-toe proportions carefully before a cut.

Facts to Know

• Hair should be cut wet.

• The best cutters cut in carefully, precisely organized sections starting with the nape of neck first to establish the point of longest length. This way the growth pattern of hair can be **STUDIED.** A precise cut grows out evenly and keeps its shape as it grows!

• The best cutters cut *moderately*, never radically—a little

off on the first go-round. If you like it and it *works* for you, more can come off on the second visit!

• Beware of the cutter who grabs a chunk of hair and "guillotines" it!

• Tip: If you are uncertain about your choice of haircutter: (1) Get to salon earlier than your appointment. Watch how he works on other clients! (2) Test him on the first go-round with a *trim*, shampoo and set, or blow-dry set.

• Is he conservative, careful, precise? Hair must be cut with careful, slow, measured sharpness, with attention to a mathematically perfect line in cleanly parted sections.

• Listen to what he has to say. Watch how he handles your hair. See if he quietly studies you standing up, to get body proportion, and sitting down, to get face proportion!

• Does he concentrate quietly? Beware of the haircutter who chats away. His attention can't be on "the job at hand!"

• A good haircutter will keep wetting hair down.

• A good haircutter keeps referring back to sections already cut as a guide.

• A good haircutter will stand you up after completing the cut to see how hair moves when *you* move. He will check for imperfect edges, an uneven or imbalanced line.

• A good haircutter will spend nearly as much time on a trim as on a major reshaping! Beware of the free-form "snip-away" technique. You're in for uneven length problems!

• Don't be afraid to share how you want your hair to look and behave with your hairstylist. Bring along pictures. Share your hair routine time and your daily routine with him. He should want to know all this. *Remember: Hair is personal!* The "cookie cutter assembly line" or the "This is what's in fashion now" approach is not for you!

• *But listen to the haircutter too!* Don't try to make your hair what it is not. If you've very curly hair, have it cut for very curly hair. Don't insist on an even, blunt, straight Greta Garbo haircut! *Don't rely on chemically straightened hair either.* Chemical straightening is unhealthy for hair and rarely looks convincing. The reverse is also true. If you have straight hair, live with it! Perms are fun for a few weeks. The possible hair damage and the growout agony isn't worth it!

BASIC LINGERIE— WARDROBE

The Perfect-Fitting Sweater-Bra

• Your everyday bra must be absolutely *smooth*, with no lace and as few seams as possible so that you can wear it under sweaters, jersey, anything thin or "clingy," as well as with most everything you own!

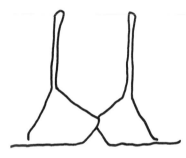

• Make sure the straps are as smooth as possible to avoid any bulge from strap adjusters.

• Try to find bras which close *in front* to avoid back bulge of hook-closure!

TRICK: Buy these everyday bras in skin color. *Skin color, not white, is the underwear neutral!* You can wear them under *everything* from black to anything knitted or sheer, and they look "invisible" (skin tone). White will separate from skin tone and show through.

• **Trick:** If you find a bra that works, instantly buy at least six—a time-saver! Bras you love have a way of "not being there" when you go back to shop for more.

• *Remember: Always match bra to skin color!* If you wear anything sheer or see-through it then becomes invisible! *NEVER* match bra to color of top! You will see the bra underneath for sure because of the contrast of skin and bra color. NEVER, ever wear a dark or black bra under a pale or see-through top. *Nothing* looks worse then to see that dark shadow underneath!

One Perfectly Fitting Smooth Strapless Bra— Skin-color to Wear Under Strapless and Any Bare Tops

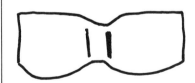

Smooth means no lace, as few seams as possible, flattest closing possible. This way you can wear it under everything from a thin jersey camisole, to a bare halter sweater, to a chiffon strapless top!

• Note: Remember, if you look, you should be able to find these bras lightweight, unconstructed, *and with the proper support for you!* There is no need for a bra to look like heavy armature.

• For maximum support a *thin* (not heavy!) plastic underwire may be necessary, but the major support is done through advances in engineering and uses of stretch fabric and molding.

• For extra smoothness and opacity, look for satiny fabrics. They are slippery so overlayers of clothing don't cling. This is especially important for evening fabrics, especially *silky* jersey!

The Pretty Bra

• Remember: Pretty lingerie can make you *feel* prettier—look for lacy, and as light and lingerie-like as you can handle!

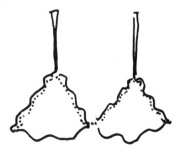

- Look for ones that are cut as *low* as possible *at the sides* for low armholes and sleeveless tops; as low as possible *in the front* so that you can wear them under your most delicate low-cut or low-buttoning tops! Front closures are best; they're smoother and lighter. **If a bit of bra does show a flash of lace peeking at the edge of a blouse** opening, it's pretty!

- Lacy bras should tone to what you are wearing. For pale or skin-toned clothes, a skin-colored lacy bra. Black lacy bras can work for black, navy, or dark brown tops.

Everyday Underpants

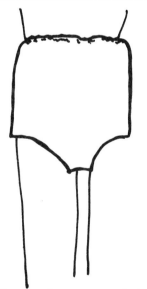

- The under-trouser briefs: From waist to top-of-leg, to wear under the thinnest or closest-fitting pants you own!

You never want to see a line of panty showing through! Or:

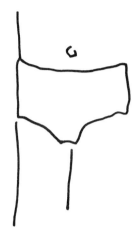

- Bikini-low with the smoothest fit over legs! To wear under trousers only if you are slim and for certain have no stomach bulge! Otherwise wear for skirts and dresses only.

- *Smooth is key*—untrimmed, flat, smooth seams!

- Always buy skin color, as it is neutral!

- Try to find underpants with a tiny bit of control if you feel you need it! Look for as sleek a surface (satiny) as possible to insure "no cling" for wearing under jersey, think silk, etc.

- **Note:** Underpants and especially those for all-day wear *should have a 100 percent cotton panel.* It breathes and is medically proven more healthful.

Pretty Panties

- "Boxer" shorts all satiny and lace-edged (matched to a bra for more delight) are best for *unclingy* dresses and skirts. Wear under pants only if they have loose pajamalike legs, or boxer shorts will bunch up and show!

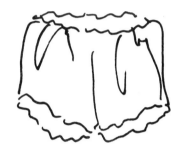

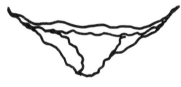

- A lacy bikini (matched to bra!) is lovely to wear under evening-dressing or any light day-dressing. Always wear underclothes made of non-clinging fabrics; otherwise check to see if the lace shows through!

Body Stocking

- Skin-toned! To wear under *anything* when you want a long smooth unbroken line: narrow knit dresses, slidey, narrow, silky ones, anything see-through—a white or pale-colored cotton gauze dress, for instance. Look for those with a little "control" in the body or a built-in bra if you need the support.

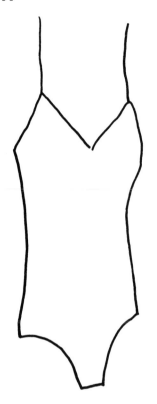

• Remember: Body stockings should not be heavy. They should be smooth and light or they defeat the purpose!

NOTE: Never wear a bra *under* a non-support body stocking. Too bulky and too many straps! Look for one that meets your figure needs.

• Color note: If you are wearing a bare black, or any dark-color, slide-of-a-dress at night (in knot or silky jersey, etc.),

wear a black body stocking. Like a bra, any edge showing through looks better if the undergarment is the same color as the dress.

Camisole (Optional)

• Nice to wear for trouser-dressing when you wear a blouse so that an edge of lace peeks through. Handy for wrap-tops that risk opening too much . . . it looks pretty to see lace! Especially handy as a layer of warmth in cold weather!

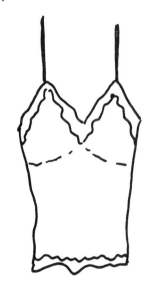

• Look for camisoles in thin, thin wool and cotton knit with lacy edges when you really need *warmth and protection!*

An alluring at-home look: a satiny or silky pajama or robe wrapped over a lacy camisole. Leave top open to waist. Just tie at waist to hold everything together!

Half-Slip

• Lacy. To wear with a button-to-hem shirtdress or skirt when you unbutton two or three bottom buttons and want the flirt of lace peeking through. Especially pretty at night! Be sure to match the slip to what you are wearing. Handy for skirts with slits if you want the same effect.

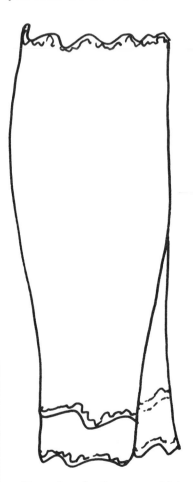

• *Very handy* for wrapskirts and wrapdresses, especially for those moments when the wrap opens—for instance, when you sit down or when a sudden breeze comes along.

TIP: If you intend to wear these under anything clingy (knit or jersey especially!), look for non-cling slips of fabric *designed to reduce static electricity!*

Slimming Trick

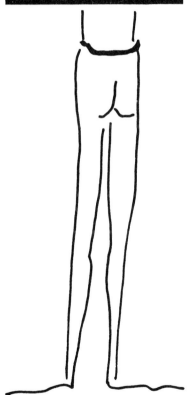

• *For ultra-slim, body-sliding clothes—Wear a seamless panty-stocking with a built-in opaque panty to insure one, long, unbroken line waist-to-toe.* No underpants or stocking

line. For more "hold" try the support kind! Even if you are slim, certain long slides-of-dresses look even better when the body is "held" a little more, for instance, thin cashmere or thin knit! Support-stretch-stockings are slicker on the surface and therefore keep clothes from clinging!
Add:

Full Slip

• Make it delicately beautiful, lacy, and luscious. Even if you don't wear it very often it's a pleasure to look at!

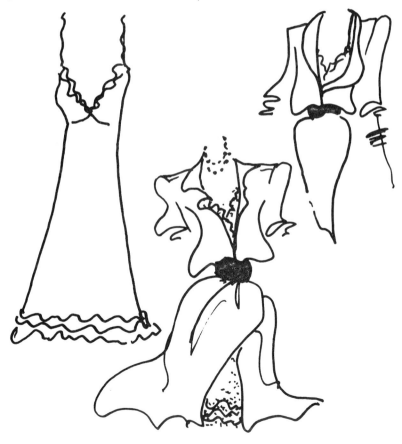

• Try to find one with a fitted top, so if you don't need a bra you can wear it over skin alone! Slide a pale wrapdress or a sheer flower-printed chiffon one over it, let a little lace show at the top, and again it will peek out when you walk!

• Extra-Feminine Look "At-Home": Wear your laciest slip under a satin kimono-wrap or a beautiful silky robe, especially if cut like a man's dressing gown—which makes a very nice contrast. A wonderful look for "dinners for two"!

SUMMER TRICKS—
Fifteen Ways To Wear a T-Shirt

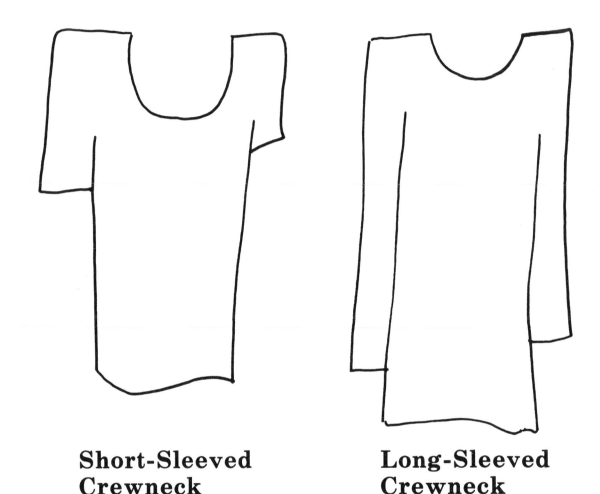

Short-Sleeved Crewneck

Long-Sleeved Crewneck

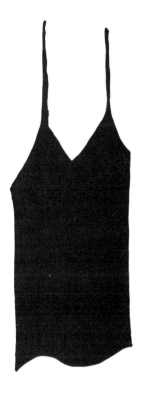

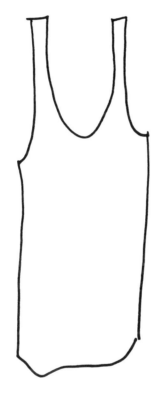

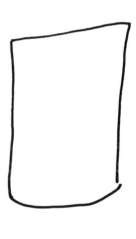

Bare
Camisole

Undershirt
Shape
(Great if you need to wear a bra as straps are wide enough to cover bra!)

Strapless
These are the shapes to collect in colors and in white!

SUMMER TRICKS

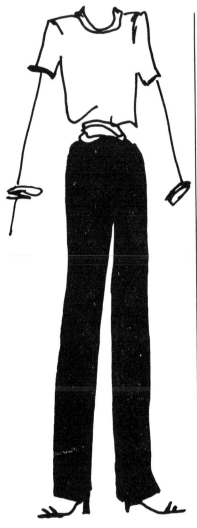

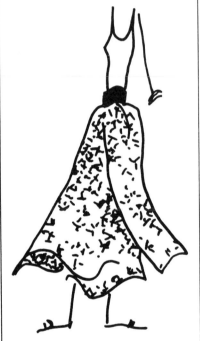

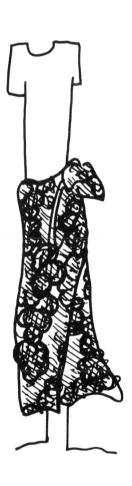

Looks

- Match a T-shirt to trousers or skirt. **City Work Day:** Navy T-shirt, navy cotton pants (or skirt), pale peanut leather belt, low-heeled peanut sandals, wood bracelets, small gold stud earrings—*plus* careful hair and makeup! Tan canvas-and-leather shoulderbag. City day, travel...A perfect summer look!

- **Country Day Version:** White T-shirt, pale blue cotton pants (or skirt), white rope-soled espadrilles, a pale washed-pink-and-blue-flower cotton scarf twisted and pulled through belt loops and short-knotted at the waist (instead of a belt!).

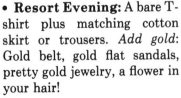

- **Resort Evening:** A bare T-shirt plus matching cotton skirt or trousers. *Add gold*: Gold belt, gold flat sandals, pretty gold jewelry, a flower in your hair!

- A T-shirt with a printed cotton sarong knotted over: quick *pretty* way to go to a **Beach-Lunch.** You can wear your bathing suit under it all! See scarf section for "How to Tie a Sarong"!

- **More Great Instant-Evening:** *Bare T-shirt plus sarong of flowered silk!* A big silk scarf or a shawl 54″ square is perfect. (Or buy a sarong-length of silk by the yard.) Belt sarong with gold belt. This will

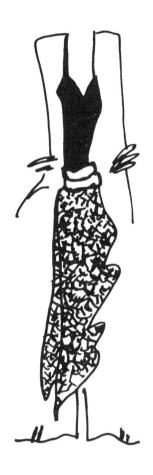

Or do a scarlet kid belt, scarlet sandals, scarlet kid tiny soft bag! *The city key: dark colors. Then you add metallic or a crayon color for accessories.* It could be a navy or brown T-shirt and pants plus gold. Try bronze metallic belt and shoes, then some pretty earrings and bracelets! *Makeup and hair are ultra important.* Or do a turnout in a pale color—pale dove, gray, palest pink, or all-white plus metallic accessories for great *Instant Resort Evening.*

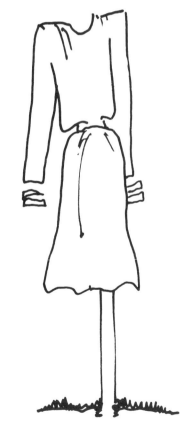

also keep it secure for the evening! Add gold sandals, pretty jewelry.

• *T-shirt and matching bottom for City Evening.* Black long-sleeved T-shirt, black silky skirt, plus gold belt, sandals and a little gold kid envelope for *City Dinner anywhere.*

• *Easy Evening:* A T-shirt and pretty print silk skirt or trousers is another version. Black tank T-shirt, red-black-and-yellow flower-printed silk skirt, gold belt and sandals. For dash (and air conditioning cover!) a big scarlet 54″ silk square over your shoulder or a scarlet cardigan sweater!

SUMMER TRICKS

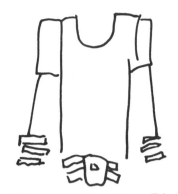

• **Summer Country Dinner!** White cotton T-shirt, gold belt, white-and-blue-check silk (or thin cotton) trousers, flat gold sandals! Some lovely bracelets . . . SUPER LOOK!

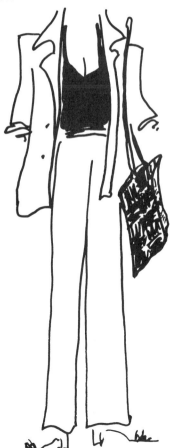

• A bare T-shirt is a pretty blouse under a cotton suit. Your old tan poplin safari jacket plus tan poplin trousers, and *a bare red T-shirt*. Belt it in peanut leather; add peanut leather sandals and you have a great *City Day* way to look and *Travel*.

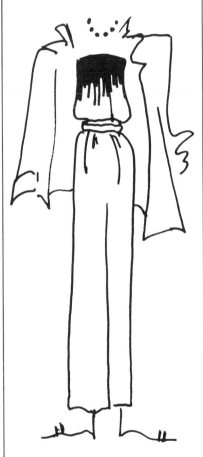

• A bare black strapless top plus safari jacket and tan trousers. Add bronze metallic belt and sandals for a quick, nice-looking way to go to an Easy Restaurant Dinner.

Great *Travel Trick:* In your carry-on bag, pack the bronze shoes, belt, tiny metallic bag, black strapless T-shirt. You are then nearly ready for dinner when you arrive! No need to unpack, and you have time for a fresh-up shower and makeup change!

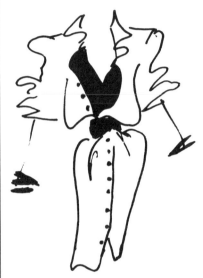

TRICK: Slide a bare camisole T-shirt in a super color under a silky or thin cotton shirtdress. *Open the dress to waist.* Add a metallic belt and sandals for *evening* or peanut leather belt and sandals for *day*! Peach camisole T-shirt under dark taupe dress; violet camisole one under navy dress! A nice way to change a look and add a dash of color!

• **How to Make an Instant Summer Suit:** Take a silk shirt ("jacket") and matching cotton pant (or skirt). Slide a

T-shirt underneath. **For *city day:*** belt and sandal in leather. **For *country:*** twist and knot a cotton scarf as a belt or use a length of hemp rope knotted at both ends to keep it from fraying! (See Belt Sec-

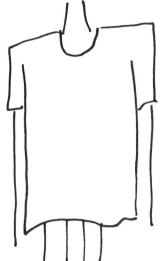

tion.) White T-shirt, navy silk shirt as jacket, navy cotton trousers. Peanut leather belt, peanut kid sandals, soft kid shoulderbag, wood and gold bracelets: *Ideal Summer Work/Day Look!*

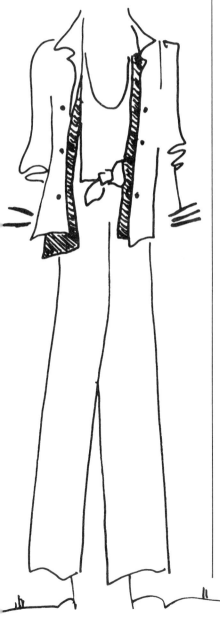

• **The Best Bathing Suit Cover:** if you have the body to carry it, is a T-shirt—especially sexy with a bikini so that you've a flash of skin between bottom of T-shirt and bikini bottom.

• *Bathing Suit Cover* for the less-perfect body: Buy a huge size man's white undershirt T-shirt. You can find these undershirts in the supermarket. Roll the sleeves; blouse and belt it with hemp rope!—It makes a fabulous short beach dress! Some people use them this way for tennis. All you add are white cotton briefs!

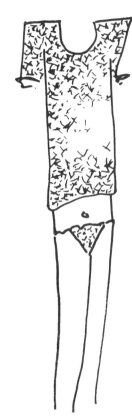

• *T-shirts: Sleep in Them!* The bigger the T-shirt the better; a giant-sized man's is perfect! On hot summer nights nothing is cooler than a white cotton T-shirt as a night cover!

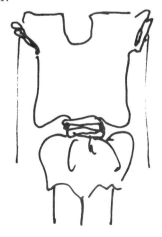

TRAVEL

The Keys to Travelling Successfully

1. Organization. Have the right tools: cases, valises, bags, etc.

2. *Preplanning.* Study where you are going, your needs, your emergency contingencies, etc.

3. Pare everything to perfect minimum. Make lists. Know your indispensables.

Have the Right Suitcases

• The best and lightest: hard frame and hard sides—soft top and bottom. The hard edges make them easier to pack as they hold their shape (don't collapse); the soft top and bottom allows for expansion.

• *Make sure they are tough.* They must stand the worst handling both from machine and man! (Have you ever seen baggage being loaded and unloaded?)

• *Make sure they are waterproof*: If you have ever received your suitcase and found it soaked through to the top three layers of clothes inside, you will know why! Tough leather, or vinyl at edges and corners, heavy-treated canvas top and bottom, or plasticized . . . even better!

• Remember: In most airports there is an acute shortage of porters. The worst surprise is what to do with your "one-ton" suitcase when there is no one around to help!

• Better pack in two smaller carry-yourself suitcases if you need to take so much! Otherwise, pare down to one small bag. (Read on for this.)

• Have a portable luggage dolly—the kind stewardesses use. You can strap it on to one of your valises! Or buy suitcases that come with attached wheels and a pull-handle.

• **Use inconspicuous luggage.** A $1,000 gorgeous leather case spells: "It's worth stealing" . . . Also, why allow anything so beautiful the horrendous wear and tear!

• **Use identifying markings,** easily seen from afar in the crush at the baggage claim area. Big yellow stickers, colored tape, bright-colored yarn knotted to handles. Make sure the ID markings are well secured so that they don't come off in the handling—or mishandling! This prevents accidental loss.

• **Never use your name and address as an ID mark.** Luggage tags should have concealed ID information flaps. Even better, put your name and *business* address on the concealed flap, *or* keep the ID *inside* the bag. Use bright markings outside to make bags easily identifiable. There are spotters at airports who love to find names and addresses of people booked out on trips. It gives them plenty of time to organize and clean out one's apartment!

• **Always lock luggage.** Keep keys in the change purse part of your wallet or somewhere safe and easily accessible. Take along an *extra set in your hand luggage* just in case you lose or misplace.

TRICK: If your suitcase is heavily packed and it's the zipper kind—or even one with snap lock—*run one or two canvas luggage belts around case for safety*. This prevents that horror of horrors—your suitcase "bursting open" on the luggage carousel; or worse, in the hold of the plane where you can't retrieve everything!

• **The best, most efficient way to travel** is with carry-on pieces only: a canvas under-the-seat duffle (with a shoulder strap) and a garment bag (with handles on both ends so that you can fold and carry it easily)! **Tip:** Call ahead to airline to check "under-seat" measure—45″ is the linear measure, but some heights and widths of seats vary occasionally!

• **TIP**: If *you check luggage, remember: Always carry in* *your hand luggage all health and beauty essentials, all valuables (jewelry, important papers, etc.), and an extra set of underwear and night clothes . . .* just in case your luggage doesn't arrive with you! Also, when you hand-carry health and beauty items there ͼless chance of spillage.

How to Pack

• **TRICK:** Plastic bags! Waste-paper basket liners for sweaters and blouses; baggies for shoes, bottles, etc.; dry-cleaner bags to slide over larger pieces of clothing *before* folding. Plastic holds air, helps cut down on creases!

• Take extra bags along—you never know when they will come in handy: for laundry, damp bathing suits, etc.

• *Roll* items such as underwear, T-shirts, night clothes. Use to stuff little gaps as you fill bag. Roll underwear *in* night clothes to keep them together in one place. Roll knits! Roll belts and socks; stuff in shoes!

• Use stockings and small items (bras, scarves, etc.) to stuff shoulders of jackets, blouses, etc.

• Always place heavy items like shoes in case first!

• Fold crushable things like silk over "cushions" of sweaters!

• Pack skirts and dresses *inside out.* If you get creases they will be inverted and will show less.

• **Trick:** Gather pants, skirts, blouses, dresses each on a thin hanger, each in a plastic cleaning bag. Lay them lengthwise in a stack across suitcase, hangers extending out on one side, hems the other. Fold hangear side over and cover with hem side—you've folded clothing into thirds. When you reach your destination, unfold, grab hangers, shake out and hang in closet. The separate plastic bags are amazing "decreasers!"

• *Learn to fold things lengthwise, in thirds.* The folds follow the "body line," minimize creases, and when you put the garment on, your shoulders, hips, etc., help fill creases out! Learn to roll uncreaseables and use to fill gaps.

• Remember the steaming-on-a-hanger-over-a-bathtub-of-hottest-water trick!

• Pack last what you will use first: night clothes, dinner dress *and* its accessories, etc.

• Pack a foldable extra duffle (the thin waterproof nylon kind!) if you have room. It is a lifesaver for those last-minute purchases!

• If you have a soft-sided valise, be sure to *pack it tightly.* This way you fill in gaps and keep clothes from creasing! (Use a smaller-sized valise if need be.)

• Always pack in an air-conditioned room in humid places. The least amount of dampness in a closed suitcase is like the rainy season in the jungle!

• *Trick to packing a garment bag:* Layer four to five garments on a single sturdy hanger. Fold one or two pairs of trousers over bar, then put skirts flat over pants, then a dress folded lengthwise down the middle. On another hanger layer blouses, four on a hanger. Button top buttons of each and stuff tissue paper in sleeves. Jackets or coats go one to a hanger over everything else. Sweaters, like pants, are lopped over the hanger bars. *This way you get the maximum amount in a bag.*

• Make a list of *everything* you pack and keep it with your passport, etc., in your handbag. *Before* leaving on a trip, check your insurance coverage. If anything is lost you have an easier time making a claim. Remember: airlines have only a very low-value coverage on loss. You will want to have your own additional insurance.

What to Pack

KEY: *Never take anything on a trip that you haven't already worn! A trip is not the place to break anything in!* If you buy new clothes for a trip, wear them first. Make sure they fit, look good, make you feel wonderful. Make sure they work with your accessories!

KEY: *Before* packing always try on anything you haven't worn for a while. Does it still fit? Does it still work? Check for open seams, a dropped hem, a stain that never came out!

• **KEY:** *Never, ever break in new shoes on a trip!* A walking tour of the Marrakech souk is no place to find out that your new flat leather sandals cut into your heels to the point of agony!

• *Planning Trick*: If you have the space in your apartment to store a folding clothes rack, buy one. *Before packing*, hang on the rack everything you plan to take. It helps you to see an overall picture so that you can make sure everything works with everything else, that you haven't eliminated any essentials or included duplicates, for example two pairs of black silk trousers when one is sufficient!

• If you don't have a hanging rack **another trick:** Lay everything out on your bed and make "scarecrows" of outfits. Check that you have essential belts, shoes, etc. Pare down, add, eliminate duplicates.

• Make lists. List all trip activities: swimming, tennis, dinner parties, black-tie dance . . . club lunches, sailing, sightseeing, meetings! Be sure to include *temperature/ weather possibilities*. If you aren't certain of the weather call ahead to the airline and check; 90° in August in Kansas City does not mean it will be the same in Paris or London.

• On a second sheet of paper, figure the *number of days you will be away*. Then start listing what you plan to wear. This is where you eventually *must become brutal*! Cross out extras. See how many combinations of looks you can make out of key pieces, etc.

• **Edit trip wardrobe to one basic color.** This means you instantly need fewer accessories. Even beauty/make-up essentials can be pared down as a result—one color nail polish, blush, etc!

• **Tip:** Use pieces that take up "no room" as color accents: scarves, shawls, thin silky jackets, blouses.

KEY: *Take with you only things you feel wonderful in . . .* you will feel better wearing them more often!

• Be sure to cut down on prints or anything that needs special accessories.

• **Trick to keeping a travel wardrobe "basic":** Make a packing plan *with shoes*. Edit them to minimize: two day shoes, one evening sandal, one slipper for beach and hotel room, one sport, touring, or walking shoe. Then plan around your shoes!

• *Jewelry*: Keep to a minimum. Take only your favorite pieces that *work* with the clothes you are taking. Remember your *Planning List*. If you plan to take **real jewelry**, keep it to the very minimum. Take only what you can wear all at once—simple gold chains, earrings, etc.

• Remember, there are cities in the U.S. and the world where parading obvious finery *only attracts trouble*! Even gold chains these days can be asking for trouble. Witness N.Y. and the gold-chain snatchers!

• *If you must take real jewelry for that major dinner*, etc., be sure to *carry it in your handbag* or keep it in the *hotel safe* when you aren't wearing it! Know that there are "eyes" who also watch those who make trips to hotel safes . . . *Be extra-careful*!

• So that you don't feel deprived ever on a trip, *after you have done all your editing* and eliminating, *add one delight—* a rose georgette blouse, a silk jacket, a slip-of-a-dress of pale apricot crepe de chine . . . three more silk 54″ squares . . . just for the joy of having them along! (See illustrated examples.)

Hand Luggage Travel Indispensables

• **Tip:** Pack beauty products, cosmetics, medicines, and vitamins in **separate bags**; add one for sun products. Nice travel splurge: Buy small *pretty* plastic-lined cotton bags. They make a hotel room look charming and *personal* when you put them around. One for medicines, one for skin, one for hair, one for makeup, one for bath/shower suppliers, one for plane—earplugs, eyemask, moisturizer, etc. *Carry them with you.*

TRICK: **To cut down on last-minute rush**, *always* keep these bags filled! *Restock* them as soon as you return home from a trip with small-sized shampoo, toothpaste, extra toothbrush, small plastic bottles of your skin cleanser, tonic, night cream, moisturiz-

er . . . packets of cold-water laundry soap, nail polish remover, your favorite skin soap in a plastic box . . . extra adhesive bandages, ponytail rubberbands, hairpins, emery boards, razor, tweezers, etc.!

• **Organize:** Make sure you have all essentials. Make a list. Start packing a few days before you leave. Keep bags open in your bedroom or bath. Whenever you remember something, *stop what you are doing, get it and pack it*! Or put it on a master list of things to buy. **Don't rely on your memory**. When you're off on a trip, the last-minute frazzle makes for easy forgetting!

TIP: *If you wear glasses*, always take along an extra pair, *plus* a copy of your prescription. *Always take along prescriptions for medicines*, etc., as customs officials could question drugs!

TIP: *Whenever you travel to any exotic place, check with your doctor.* Are there prevention medicines or immunizations you should have? Allow time for immunizations, as some have to be spaced over a few weeks.

• **Handy Checklist: For Hand Luggage:** Address book, bottle opener, scissors, face cloth, eyedrops, hand cream, shower cap, small mag-

nifying mirror and tweezers, earplugs and eyemask (if you use them), folding umbrella, thin folding raincoat (small enough to stash in handbag!), thin rubber rain booties (These could be your treasure of the trip!), tiny sewing kit, stick of spot remover, small alarm clock.

TIP: Always organize these items by category in separate cases—cotton bags, nylon ones, even plastic sandwich bags!

• **Organize your handbag.** A shoulder bag is best. When traveling it is helpful to have hands free for tickets, tips, carrying luggage . . . and safer too!

• *Make sure everything you need fits into your bag comfortably.* Test it! If you are buying a new bag, *test it* in the store.

• Make sure your handbag isn't too heavy. Check *all* carry-on luggage for weight! There is nothing worse than a "dislocated shoulder" before you even board the plane. Does the bag balance correctly? Are you taking too much? See "Handbag Section."

• *Tip*: Do not **put passport, travelers checks, tickets, credit cards, etc., into one**

holder! *Keep them separate* from one another! This way if you lose one you don't lose everything!

- **Handbag Checklist:**

- Passport

- Plane ticket

- Travelers checks—Tip: Keep travelers checks numbers separate from checks. **Give a copy to a friend reachable at home!**

- Tickets of any kind (train, boat, etc.)

- Wallet/money

- Extra Wallet for foreign currency. Remember, most foreign currency, including coins, is larger than American!

- Credit card case

- Glasses

- Dark glasses

- Tissues

- Pillbox (Dramamine, aspirin, etc.)

- Map and guides

- Pad and pens

- Jewelry roll (for real jewelry)

- Extra passport pictures for last-minute visas (or if you lose your passport!)

To Have in Handbag or Carry-on Bag—Planes

- Moisturizer, handcream, and lip cream (gloss, Chapstick, etc.) Remember: the pressurized cabins are dry climates and are dehydrating! You will feel amazingly better if you apply moisturizer several times during your trip.

- A small mineral water spray is a fabulous face refresher and hydrating as well! **Tip:** Wear the smallest amount of makeup possible at beginning of plane trip, just enough to get you aboard looking pulled-together—a bit of cheek color, some gloss, a dash of eyeshadow, a moisturizer instead of foundation. *Do your makeup on arrival!*

- *Toothbrush and toothpaste*: a reviver, especially if you nap!

- *A silk or cotton scarf*: to protect head or neck from airplane air-conditioning drafts or to use as an eye shade to sleep . . . AND if your hair looks worn out at the end of a long trip, wrap a neat head turban around it! Do fresh makeup and you look revived!

- Eyedrops: eyes get strained from reading as well as the dry plane climate!

- *Cologne*: spray your favorite anytime you need a *pickup*. It also makes your "environment" smell delicious!

- Aspirin, vitamins, etc., in a pillbox.

- **Travel essentials:** Your blanket-shawl (see scarf/shawl section) to keep you cozy, to use as thin cardigan sweater for drafts, to sleep under, to fold and use as an **extra pillow!**

- *To pass the time*: Bring along a favorite book, letter paper, and envelopes. Plane time is *great* to use to catch up on letters owed or to rewrite address book!

- **On board:** Wear your most comfortable shoes or sandals. Try to wear them a little on the loose side in case of foot-swelling.

- *Walk around the cabin regularly*. Stretch your legs. Stretch! Sitting for a whole trip is fatiguing; muscles cramp; circulation is constricted. *It is not healthy!*

TIP: On plane trips *eat lightly, drink a lot of water*. Remember, plane cabin dryness is dehydrating! Keep alcohol to a minimum! Alcohol constricts blood vessels and cuts down circulation, which is exactly what you want to avoid!

Car Travel

- A small pillow and thin blanket are handy for napping.

- Keep a case of beauty essentials nearby, plus:

- Cologne for a reviving spray

- A small mineral water spray to cleanse your face, rehydrate, and wake you up!

- Hand cream. Give your hands a treatment! If you are doing the driving put on a good slather of cream, then some old leather gloves so your hands don't slide on the wheel! If you *are not driving* use hand cream plus thin cotton gloves.

- Tissues

- Eyedrops for eyestrain

- Dark glasses

- A scarf to keep hair from blowing if windows are open, to keep draft off if air conditioning is on!

- Notepaper and pens (for thoughts)

- A small container with change for tolls!

- A thermos of spring water and a cup—for aspirin, car sickness pills, etc.

- Remember, when car traveling *stop often, get out and walk around.* Stretch your legs—even "jog" around a little to get circulation going. This is the best reviver and a lot healthier than coffee!

- Instead of packing crushables in a valise, take advantage of trunk space: lay them flat with a plastic protector on top.

- **TIP:** For long car trips, especially in untrafficked areas, a *C.B. radio is essential!* As well as supplying local weather information and directions, it's a safety measure: In case of breakdowns, accidents or any trouble you can get help fast!

WHEN YOU GET TO YOUR DESTINATION

- **Tip for charm in hotel rooms:** (1) Your favorite room spray or a small box of potpourri, for a nice, homey smell! (2) A folding picture frame with photos of your "friendliest faces." (3) Throw your pretty scarves and shawls over chairs and at the foot of your bed instead of putting them into drawers! (4) Buy fresh flowers when you arrive. Put them in the bathroom, too! Three small roses in a glass can make a world of difference! (5) Line your suitcase with scented flannels or scented paper before packing. When you remove your clothes you will be wafted with delicious smells!

Tips on Travel Dressing

- "Dress comfortably" does not mean throw on your old red pullover and a pair of jeans! (Unless you're flying from one farm to another!)

- Key: *You want to "fit in" when you arrive*—especially if you are traveling to a city!

A SUIT IS THE BEST BET! (1) A jacket and matching easy, "sitable" skirt or trousers. (2) A fabric that is *minimally* crushable (jersey, thin gabardine, poplin, knit, thin cotton canvas or twill when you are going to hot climates). (3) **To wear with suit:** a pullover of knit or cotton string or a blouse. **Key:** If you tone all of this to your packed wardrobe, you've got *extra pieces* to play with! (4) Throw your knitted or thin wool shawl over your shoulder. (5) Add a raincoat (or "proper" coat if you are going to cold climates) and you are set. (6) Make sure that your accessories are toned to what you are packing. Your traveling bag is then your day bag; the shoes you are wearing are an extra pair of shoes. (They could be your "comfortable walking shoes" for the trip!)

TRAVEL

Perfect for travel to New York, Paris, London, Chicago, San Francisco, Montreal, etc.

Use Basic Wardrobe Section as a guide.

Best fabrics for travel: Jersey: Fall/Winter/Spring. For summer, substitute linen blends, blends of cotton/silk, cotton poplin, etc. Sweaters and wool knit become cotton string or knit for summer. Shawls: wool-and-silk ones work winter and summer; rayon ones are seasonless.

BASIC WORKOUT COLOR: Beige. A good travel neutral could also be navy, gray, taupe, etc.!

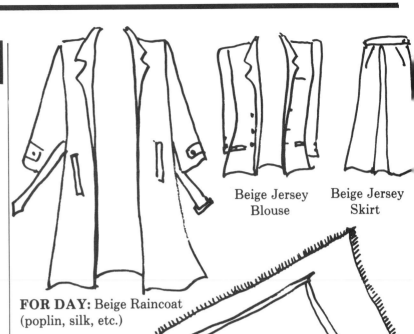

Beige Jersey Blouse

Beige Jersey Skirt

FOR DAY: Beige Raincoat (poplin, silk, etc.)

Beige Blanket-Shawl in Cashmere Knit or Challis or Alpaca and Wool
1 Peach Silk 54″ Square (for pretty evening touch!)

Peanut Leather Shoulderbag
Peanut Leather **Small** Bag (Use inside big one or alone for restaurant or easy eve!)

Peanut Leather "Skirt" Shoe
Peanut Leather Walking Shoe (sturdy enough to take rain!)

KEEP ACCESSORIES TO ONE NEUTRAL

Peanut Leather Belt
Dark Beige Suede Belt/Gold Buckle

KEEP EVENING ACCESSORIES TO ONE COLOR: GOLD:

Add: One Long *Pale* Beige Matte Jersey Dress belt in Gold. Add Gold Sandals, pretty jewels, beige shawl = Important Evening

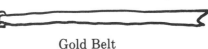

Gold Sandal   Gold Bag   Gold Belt

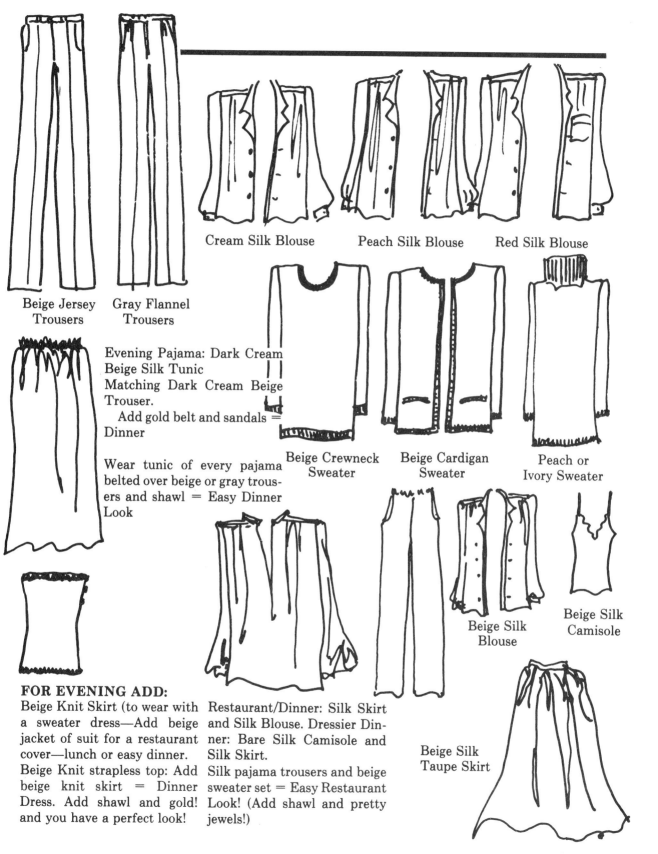

Beige Jersey
Trousers

Gray Flannel
Trousers

Cream Silk Blouse

Peach Silk Blouse

Red Silk Blouse

Evening Pajama: Dark Cream
Beige Silk Tunic
Matching Dark Cream Beige
Trouser.
 Add gold belt and sandals =
Dinner

Wear tunic of every pajama
belted over beige or gray trousers and shawl = Easy Dinner
Look

Beige Crewneck
Sweater

Beige Cardigan
Sweater

Peach or
Ivory Sweater

Beige Silk
Blouse

Beige Silk
Camisole

FOR EVENING ADD:
Beige Knit Skirt (to wear with
a sweater dress—Add beige
jacket of suit for a restaurant
cover—lunch or easy dinner.
Beige Knit strapless top: Add
beige knit skirt = Dinner
Dress. Add shawl and gold!
and you have a perfect look!

Restaurant/Dinner: Silk Skirt
and Silk Blouse. Dressier Dinner: Bare Silk Camisole and
Silk Skirt.
Silk pajama trousers and beige
sweater set = Easy Restaurant
Look! (Add shawl and pretty
jewels!)

Beige Silk
Taupe Skirt

TRAVEL

• For city travel you will need at least *two looks for restaurant dinners*: dresses or tops and skirts that look like dresses.

Think dark, medium or neutral tones.

Think silky soft fabrics, ones that are both packable *and* pretty to wear! Save pale pink silk for a *hot* resort trip!

• Reminder: Comfortable day shoes, and be sure they are broken in *before* trip!

TIP: Key to city dressing, winter or summer—*basic neutral colors*: black, navy, gray, beige. **Use color as *accents*:** a blouse, jacket, scarf, shawl.

• *Fabrics for Basic Big City Summer*: Think linen blends, cotton and silk instead of wool and jersey.

• **Summer City Essential:** Comfortable *walking sandals* with a bit of a heel.

• **City Travel Reminder** for Any Season: *Thin* raincoat—silk, thin treated cotton—plus folding umbrella.

• **Hot City Dressing Tip:** If it's in the 90s, even *silk* may be too hot! Thin, *dark cotton* and *loose caftan dress shapes* are coolest—no binding of waist as with skirts, no extra layers of tops, no covered legs as with trousers! See Basic Dress Guide for shapes. The coolest are loose from shoulder to hem, thereby creating an air-space between body and fabric: "built-in" air conditioning!

• *Tip: For any city evening where "table-life" is a part of the routine* . . . i.e., dinners, meetings, lunches, (conventions, business trips, etc.) . . . pretty touches that show *over* the table are key: earrings, scarves, necklaces. A bare dinner dress with a thin jacket as a covering looks wonderful across the table!

• Tip: *Europe City Travel Summer and Winter: Milan, London, Paris, and Munich can be cold and rainy*! Be sure to be prepared with proper rain gear *and* additional layers of warmth: a few more pullovers, woolly shawls, a lining that buttons into raincoat (in fur or alpaca), gloves, warm nightclothes, even socks to sleep in!

• **Tip for *Paris and Milan*:** one *dresses up more in evening*! For restaurants: short, feminine, even bare dresses (with a silky jacket or shawl) plus pretty jewelry!

• *New York* **is a bit less dressy:** silk trousers and a pretty sweater or a suit with a strapless camisole . . .

• *Rome* **is a southern city!** One sees more *color here*. For nights: Bright silky bare blouses, pajamas . . . pastels in hot summer! In winter stick to proper city dressing and city neutral colors.

• *San Francisco and Chicago* **are more conservative** than New York. See dress section for covered dinner dresses, two-piece jersey dresses for day. One wears trousers less. **These cities are even cool in summer!** Bring one warm covering —blanket-shawl is ideal!

• *Los Angeles*: **Day:** Easy trouser-dressing looks (pants and pretty pullovers). **Night:** Easy sexy looks (like Rome!)— pajamas, beautiful shirts, silk pants, bare tops, bright ankle skirts in summer. Crepe de chine pants, silk skirts, and bare tops are always perfect.

Basic Travel Wardrobe— Guideline
Basic Resort: Hot

• **Key: The usual rule:** tone everything so that everything works well together!

TWO BATHING SUITS

One or two Beach Covers. A big white caftan for hot places *or* a cozy brushed

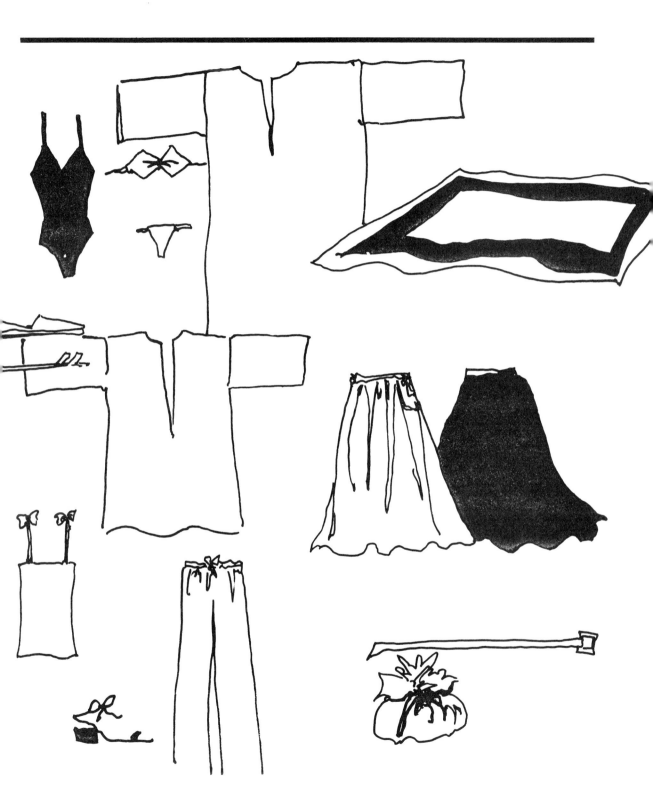

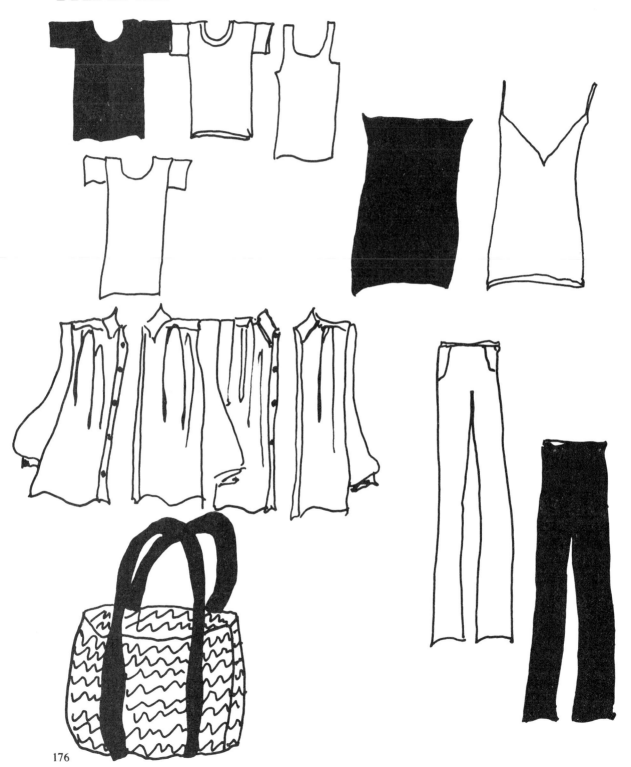

176

cotton long pullover for cool places.

Espadrilles

Stack of silk and cotton scarves to use as belts, bras, head covers, sarongs, evening coverings, etc.!

One evening cover (a thin wool or silk shawl or big silky "jacket")

T-shirts and cotton shirts . . . 4–6

Two Bare T-shirts (camisoles and strapless) to wear with skirts for easy evening! And day (with trousers.)

One Pair of pale cotton trousers (white, cream)

One Pair of dark cotton trousers (navy or tan)

One Jacket (to match light or dark trouser)

One Night sandal

One Soft Pale cotton day skirt (white, cream)
One Soft dark cotton day skirt (navy, tan)

1 Dinner pajama. Silk or crepe de chine pants and matching blouse and/or matching bare top.

TIP: *The hotter the place,*

the colder the air conditioning can be! Be prepared with a thin wool shawl, thin cotton cardigan, or sweater/kimono jacket of white knitted cashmere.

• *Palm Beach:* white, pales, sea colors (reds, cobalt blues, wonderful clean colors that look fabulous in the sun!), cotton knit T-shirt dresses, gauze cotton and cotton-shirting sundresses, big loose cotton shirtdresses. *Add white sandals, a straw Panama for a great lunch look!* The look of trim white trousers and a white shirt or white T-shirt is perfect! **Evening: dressy:** Think boat cruises . . . printed georgette pajamas, a long white silk bare dress to wear with gold sandals, a gorgeously colored silk caftan to the floor—extra pretty looks! Remember to bring high-heeled gold sandals and gold accessories for evening.

• *Islands—Caribbean:* *Beach colors, white!* T-shirt dresses, gauze skirts and tops, loose dresses of gauze and crinkly cotton, thin cotton trousers and big white gauze shirts (cut like a man's). Add a Panama straw hat (sun!). *Loose* bathing suit covers are cooler! Sarongs! A big Moroccan caftan to the ankle of pale cotton or white cotton gauze (cool and easy and chic!). **Nights:** silky caftans, paja-

mas, long gauze or silky skirts and bare pretty tops. Add a blanket-shawl as it can be a cool night. White cashmere or thin wool are perfect day or night! Acapulco, etc., has same requirements as islands.

• *Mediterranean:* South of France, Italian Beach Resorts, etc. Sun colors, white! Navy (sailing colors)! as there is a big boat life around the Mediterranean. White cotton T-shirt and white pants could be a uniform! Add navy sailing sweater or navy cashmere knitted shawl for cool evenings in a seaside outdoor restaurant. Sarongs and big cotton caftans, bikinis, and monokinis, espadrilles. **Pretty, sexy evening:** long gauzy skirts, bare tops, silk shirts and white silk pants with gold sandals! Especially in Mediterranean places, check out the look that is "In" . . . there is always a new one! It could be a certain big cotton shirt, a sarong wrapskirt, a giant white sweatshirt, whatever. You may want to join in.

• **Extras:** For places where one dresses at night, take high-heeled sandals, a pretty bag for night (gold)!, plus extra silk shawl for evening cover! Add pretty evening bits: strapless and bare camisoles, floaty chiffon pajama or tunics to wear over silk pants, one or two bare, silky, floaty dresses, one dinner dress (short, silky restaurant-looking . . . see city summer trip wardrobe and dresses section). Remember, silk folds to nothing, takes no room!

• If you are a "beach" person, add:

• More bathing suits

• One or two more thin beach covers (for *hot* resorts)

• One thin cotton peasant skirt to wear for beach walks!

• Straw hat for protection (or buy one on arrival!)

• Cotton shorts (white ones can double for tennis!)

Cruises

Use the preceding lists for Resort Dressing. **Note: Evening plays a big part in cruise life.** Count the number of days you will be on board and plan from there. See "Palm Beach" for evening suggestions.
TIP: No matter how far south you are sailing, *nights on board ship can be cool;* days too! **Take one warm day cover** (big sweater, white cashmere blanket/shawl and **one for evening!**)

Basic Resort: Cool

(Maine, Washington, North-west mountains, Canada in summer) **TIP:** *Country classic!* Remember to tone everything!

Jeans

Long sleeved T-shirts

Windbreaker jacket (rainproof)

Sweaters—One heavy (Irish knit!) pullover, one regular pullover and matching cardigan

One Corduroy pants or jeans

One Gray-flannel pants

One Pretty blouse or silky tunic top to wear at night

Moccasins or sneakers and *warm* socks!

One pretty cotton skirt for day.
A jeans skirt or tan cotton poplin one. Shorts—it often gets hot in the daytime.

Warm bathing suit cover

Two bathing suits

T-shirts.
Cotton shirts

Two cotton pants (tan, navy)

Safari shirt . . . always.

Cotton squares all sizes

Thin cotton robe

Espadrilles
Day sandals
Night sandals (gold)
Cashmere or flannel shawl!
Add: **1 Easy pretty evening look—navy silk pajama** for example.

Guideline for a Four-to-five Day or Long Weekend in the Sun

• **TIP:** If this is the kind of vacation break you take often—an escape three or four times in the winter to an island, or every weekend or two in the summer—**keep all these pieces in one part of closet, clean and ready to go!**
Have on hand:

• One Duffle Bag (carry-on plane size)

• In it pack:
Two bathing suits

Three white shirts (one silk, two cotton)
One "big" cotton work-shirt—a man's faded-blue oxford or a well-washed blue-and-white-striped cotton to wear with pants, shorts . . . *big enough* to wear over a bathing suit!

One loose, white thin cotton shirtdress to wear daytime, over bathing suit, etc.!

One white wool cardigan

White cotton pants

White cotton shorts

Navy cotton pants

One thin cotton *full* skirt—a color or print—to *midcalf plus* a *bare top.*

One pajama (thin silky trouser and matching tunic or kimono top to wrap over)—in flattering a color!

One white T-shirt, one navy T-shirt, one white *bare* T-shirt.

Flat gold sandals

Espadrilles

One tiny gold kid evening bag for dash, for day too! Three belts: white canvas, gold kid, one hemp rope.

White, thin cotton kimono plus thin nightgown.

Trick for travel: *Wear* on plane (Train or Car!) an easy, seasonless look

Tan poplin or gabardine

pants or tan wrapskirt

Tan jacket (shirt-jacket or safari-jacket shape)

Cotton shirt

Shoe: tan woven leather moccasin

Tan canvas and leather inside bag:

• Jewelry: Gold neck chain, gold cuffs. Wear gold hoop earrings on plane. That's all!

If you are flying from cold climate to hot weekend

• *Under* jacket: Wear one or two sweaters *over* cotton shirt—a cardigan and a pullover for example!

• *Under* cotton pants: wear wool socks and thermal underpants over regular ones! (Wear ribbed, woolly tights under skirt.) Of course this all depends on the degree of cold.

• **Strip down on plane!** Tuck socks and "woollies" into duffle, tie cardigan around your waist, put pullover *into* duffle, and jacket on your arm. You arrive dressed in a cotton shirt and cotton pants (or a shirt and skirt)—**cool and perfect!**

Work-out

White cotton kimono bathrobe + a bathing suit = Pretty Beach Cover

White shirtdress + belt + es-

padrilles = Day Town

White shirtdress open over bikini top + gold belt + gold sandals = Pretty Lunch Look beachside or drinks!

White silk shirt + shorts + gold sandals + gold belt = Super Lunch Look!

White silk shirt knotted over white pants + gold = drinks

White *cotton* shirt + white pants + espadrilles = Sailing (white sweater over shoulders or knotted around waist)

White cotton skirt + navy pants + espadrilles = Day Bicycling, Picnic, etc.

White cotton shirt knotted over peasant skirt + gold = Drink, Pretty Evening

Bare white T-shirt + shorts = Tennis

Bare white T-shirt + silky pants + gold = Drinks

Pajama = Dinner Party

Bare top + skirt + gold = Dancing

Big man's faded shirt + shorts + espadrilles = After-breakfast walk

Big man's faded shirt + bathing suit = Beach Cover.

WEATHER DRESSIN

Guidelines

The following lists are *practical essentials* to know about when dealing with extremes of temperature and weather. AND THEY WORK!

Hot-Weather Tips

• *Loose dresses* (loose from shoulder to hem) *are coolest!* Remember the style of desert Arabs: caftans, loose flowing robes!

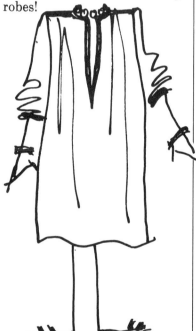

• **For** *day-city:* Dresses of thin cotton, cotton knit, thin linen and cotton (rather than silk!) are more absorbent, less sticky, therefore cooler.

• **For** *day-resort:* Gauzy caftans and big, loose shapes that fall to the ankle! Try it:

The "tent" of fabric creates an air space . . . a breeze! Built-in air conditioning! **Another way:** Big, loose "men's" shirts over loose drawstring cotton pants (like Indian and Mexican men wear!)

• *The lighter the color, the more heat reflection, the cooler!* As white is *too* un-city, wear *pale beige*. In hot resorts wear WHITE—nothing looks better in the sun! **General Rule:** Think of white and sand colors. They are the coolest and look perfect anywhere!

• **Wear cotton underwear!** It's cooler *and* healthier!

• **Remember:** *Bare* **feet and sandals** can be killing in hot weather! For days when it's extra-hot make sure you wear your most "broken-in" shoes. Slip some extra adhesive bandages, a small tin of talcum or foot powder in your bag if you plan a day of walking—especially in the city!

• **Evening:** *Loose* tunics and *thin* silky or gauzy pants, loose pretty tops, gauzy ankleskirts are airy and cool!

• **Collect T-shirts:** big, loose, tunic-y oversized ones; bare ones, classic shapes! They are ideal and cool!

• **Keep jewelry to a minimum.** Rely on earrings. When it's really hot, bracelets and necklaces look hot, feel worse!

• **Hair:** Keep hair well off face and neck. It looks and feels better! *Wear cotton head scarves* in the day. They absorb perspiration, feel cooler!

Cold-Weather Tips

• *Essentials to have*: Storm boots are indispensable, warm *furry, WATERPROOF* ones!

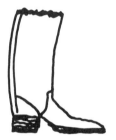

• **Tip:** Always buy them one size larger so that you can wear wool socks underneath! Remember, for warmth toes must have airspace. Tight boots are colder!

• **Tip:** Wear a pair of 100 percent silk socks *under* your wool ones . . . true insulation! *Men's silk* evening socks may be the answer if you can't find women's.

• *For protection on coldest days*: thin *silk undershirts* and silk thigh-long *underpants* or *thermal underwear!* Wear them under everything (even a business meeting turnout)! Who's to know?

• *Silk or silk-lined gloves* to wear *under wool* or leather ones for insulation!

• Woolly ribbed tights. Wear a thin layer of silk underwear underneath for more insulation!

• *For cold days when there is no wet weather*: Walking shoes with an *all-crepe sole* and heel keep you insulated from frozen pavement! *Remember the one-size-larger tip* so that you can wear them with woolly stockings. Then you can slip in a pair of THERMAL INSOLES to make shoes smaller if you wear them with a thinner stocking. The thermal insole means more protection!

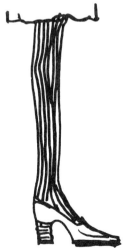

• *A rainproof coat* with an extra warm lining: fur, alpaca, or

down. The furry, cozy lining next to your body is warmest!

• *A knitted wool hat* (a watch cap!) worn *under* a thin wool or silk or cashmere kerchief is about the warmest, most protective head cover combination.

• *Real down coats or vests!* Wear a layer of silk and one of thin wool underneath—there is nothing lighter or warmer! **Remember:** *several thin layers are warmer than one heavy one!*

• *Shearling coats and jackets are ultra warm.* You have fur next to the body, and a light and totally wind-resistant skin against the weather!

• *Mufflers keep your neck and chest protected and warm!* **Tip: Neck, chest, ears, hands, top of head, rib cage, and feet (the extremities, etc.) are the target areas to protect!** They lose body warmth fastest.

Wet-Weather Tips: Essentials That Work!

• *Rain Boots*: The real waterproof ones that enable you to stand in a puddle for hours and have dry feet! **Tip:** Wear a thin cotton sock underneath, as the rubber or plastic boots do not breathe and cotton absorbs perspiration!

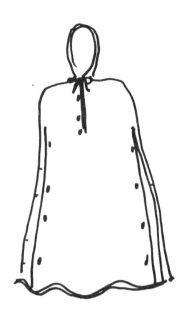

• *A big waterproof rain poncho*—the thin nylon kind from the L. L. Bean catalog or riding shops! Perfect to wear *over everything* from fur coats to a thin silk dress in summer! The one that comes with an attached hood gives the best protection, and you can fold it into a shopping/tote bag!

• *Collapsible* rain umbrella (man-sized) fits perfectly into a day shoulder tote for "it-may-rain-days."

• A big rainproof *zipper* shoulder tote (thin nylon type folds to nothing). Put it in your handbag on an "ify" day and put your expensive leather handbag IN IT for rain protection! The zipper is important for complete protection of your fragile items!

MATERNITY DRESSING

Basic Wardrobe

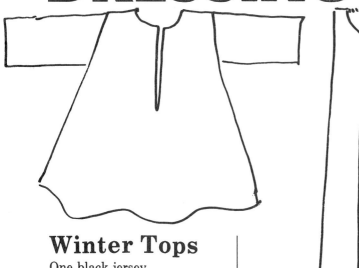

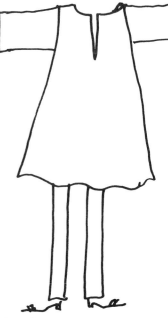

Winter Tops

One black jersey

One navy jersey

One bordeaux silk

One black silk

Two white silk (or one cream and one white to wear *under* the darks for a bit of light!)

One dark rosy lavender silk (Wear over any of pants above for evening.)

Scarlet silk (Wear for evening alone over pants or *under jersey tops* to add dash for day!)

One taupe knitted lambswool or cashmere top—your sweater! (Wear a silk tunic with any pair of trousers above.)

Pants

One black jersey

One navy jersey

One black silk

One bordeaux silk

Dark taupe jersey, wool crepe, or knit

Caftan Dress (Short)

One dark jersey for winter (to wear with dark pair of trousers and matching shoe)
One shirting cotton (i.e., a thin *vertical* stripe on white)
One navy crinkle cotton for summer *hot* day—the coolest for country and city!

Summer Tops

One thin navy cotton

One thin red cotton

One dark sand

Two thin white cotton

Pants

One navy cotton
One black cotton
One dark tan cotton
One white cotton for hot climates
Remember, the winter silks work for summer too!

Evening

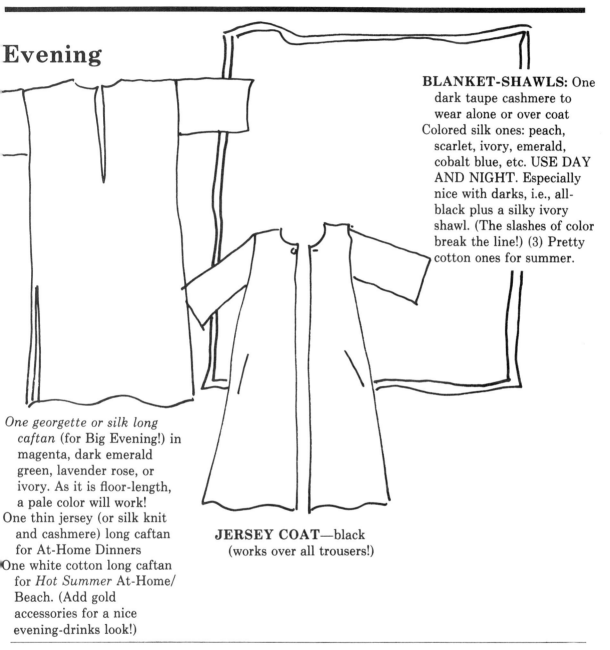

BLANKET-SHAWLS: One dark taupe cashmere to wear alone or over coat
Colored silk ones: peach, scarlet, ivory, emerald, cobalt blue, etc. USE DAY AND NIGHT. Especially nice with darks, i.e., all-black plus a silky ivory shawl. (The slashes of color break the line!) (3) Pretty cotton ones for summer.

One georgette or silk long caftan (for Big Evening!) in magenta, dark emerald green, lavender rose, or ivory. As it is floor-length, a pale color will work!
One thin jersey (or silk knit and cashmere) long caftan for At-Home Dinners
One white cotton long caftan for *Hot Summer* At-Home/ Beach. (Add gold accessories for a nice evening-drinks look!)

JERSEY COAT—black
(works over all trousers!)

Shoes

Day: peanut

Day/Eve: black, scarlet, peanut, gold sandals

Evening: gold, black satin

MATERNITY DRESSING

• **Note: this is the ideal, good-looking camouflage wardrobe for overweight problems!** If you are overweight, you will find helpful guides.

The key to successful and attractive maternity dressing:

• Always: *Wonderful hair* well off the shoulders and self-manageable! Have hair cut and conditioned regularly!.

Wear *perfect makeup* all the time. It is psychologically important! It makes you feel better as well as look better!

• *Always perfect hands and feet.* This means *regular manicures and pedicures!* It's **psychologically** uplifting!

• **WARDROBE: The basic pieces:** (1) Tunic tops mid-thigh long—never shorter! (2) Narrow-legged pants. (3) Caftan shapes as dresses with length just below the knee or floor-length for evening.

• **Tip: Tunic tops should fit in shoulders.** They work best **cut on the *bias*.** This way fabric will fall gracefully over the stomach no matter how big it becomes. **Never wear shapes that are too constructed—they are bulky! Key:** untailored and soft!

• **Think solid colors!** All pieces will work better together, interchange and LOOK better (less "remarkable").

• **Think dark, basic tones.** Remember, light tones attract the eye . . . and enlarge! Dark tones minimize. *Use color in accessories:* pretty shoes, shawls, scarves, jewelry. You want to draw the eye away from the bulky part and toward the extremities!

• **Think *soft fabrics*.** Stiff fabrics don't fall gracefully. **IDEAL:** Wool jersey for winter and cotton jersey for summer, matte jersey, silk jersey. **Think *floaty fabrics*.**

• **Key: *Thin* layers add less bulk.** When you are pregnant you sometimes tend to feel warm and claustrophobic. Even in winter, a wool jersey kimono-coat with a big cashmere or flannel/wool blanket-shawl—or another layer of a wool jersey poncho or unlined soft *cape—on top* are as warm as a single, heavy coat *and softer, more attractive, more figure-flattering!*

• **Tip: Remember the trick of *toning legs and feet*** if you aren't wearing *narrow pants!* The *long leg line* is what you want to create to detract from and balance the bulky part!

• **Tip: If you are wearing a** dress, *length is key!* Too long is draggy, too short is top-heavy. The skirt length area to work around is just covering the knee.

• **Tip: Keep shoes *delicate, pretty, and low-heeled*.** You will feel steadier, more balanced and comfortable. You *need* careful balance!

• **Think shoes in colors—** red, gold, green, purple . . . especially when you are wearing pants! A dark trouser creates a long leg-line. A bright green sandal with pretty feet, toe nails painted scarlet, can look and feel wonderful! Also, remember that when you are pregnant, feet tend to swell. Be prepared with comfortable, well-fitting, roomy shoes!

• **Key: *Narrow*-legged pants!** No matter what the fashion, remember, you are trying to balance bulk and create a long, lean line . . . *a narrow leg is key!*

• **Remember: Keep exercising.** Follow your doctor's directions as to what kind of exercise and how long, but *do exercise* every day *regularly!* (1) You will stay in shape longer. (2) You will get back in shape faster. (3) Medical evidence indicates that exercise helps release tension, reduce anxiety, prevent depression!

- **Guideline: Basic maternity wardrobe** (for hot and cold weather). *Note*: All tops are planned to work with all bottoms, which means endless looks!

- Note: There are **more items** per shape listed in wardrobe than usual, tunics and shoes, for example! **Reason:** You will want as many pleasures and delights as you can afford for personal cheer, as well as attractive dressing touches, to counterbalance the emotional and physical changes you are dealing with.

- **Fabric Tip:** Stay with *natural* (as opposed to man-made) *fibers* if you can: wool, silk, cotton. Natural fibers tend to breathe more, and when your body begins to change biologically this is a key to comfort.

- *Beach tricks Cover-Ups:* Huge, oversized, loose men's shirts to mid-thigh! Roll the sleeves. Wear with straw sandals, a big straw hat, and shoulder basket:

Mexican men's white cotton shirts, the Brooks Brothers variety in white or striped cotton, or Indian tunics called "Kurtas" in thin cotton. These are often delicately embroidered in white, they come in **wonderful colors** and solid white cotton, *and* they also come in *thin silk for evening— A great look on the beach* with bare legs or over thin, cotton trousers!

Look for Arab djellabahs, Moroccan men's caftans, in ethnic shops (especially in white cotton or pale shirting stripes). They are ideal for at-home dinners or an easy, private evening! *Remember, always think oversized.*

DIET TIPS

The best and safest diet is to count calories. Eat a balanced menu with a clearly defined calorie limit. It may take longer than a crash diet but is healthier and longer-lasting. Slower weight loss means the body has time to adjust, which means the weight is easier to keep off!

1. Keep a calorie counter:

- In your handbag

- In your kitchen

- Next to your bed!

Refer to it constantly. At night in bed, when you are just about to turn off the lights and you get that "chocolate chip craving!" *Read the calorie counter.* Psychologically seeing those numbers helps end the craving fast.

2. Keep pictures around (especially in the kitchen) of slim, great-looking people plus one fat one. Sounds "demented," but take the time to look at them just before you stuff the bread and butter in your mouth!

3. If you have a family who are not dieting: At meals do the serving in the kitchen—not at the table. This way you won't be tempted for a "tiny" helping of whipped potatoes . . .

4. If you don't have a family, *clean up your kitchen!* Keep the shelves and refrigerator bare of any possible temptations. Spartan bare! This way, when you have a craving that no psychological trick can assuage, you have no butter, no bread, no cookies, no honey, no bars of chocolate hidden away. What good is a spoonful of vinegar when you want brownies! To Do: Keep on hand lots of bottled water, skimmed milk for coffee, tons of fresh raw vegetables (carrots, cucumbers, celery, etc.), fresh fruit (but low-calorie ones; a big apple can be over a

DIET TIPS

hundred calories!) white meat chickens, turkey, thin bran biscuits, etc.

Tip: Always clean fruit when you buy it. Also vegetables. Cut them up and store in a huge bowl covered by a damp towel (to keep them crisp!) in your refrigerator. This way they are there when you need to munch on something.

Tip: Don't be fooled by health food store products. They may *sound* slimming, but read the calorie count on the labels first. *Get into the habit of reading all food labels.* One bran/wheat biscuit versus another can vary in number of calories . . . five calories add up quickly to a hundred!

The point: A calorie "bank" is what you must think of. Saving 5–10 calories in one place means you can afford more at another meal!

Tip:—Restaurants/Dinner Parties: When you are going to a restaurant or to dinner at a private home, be spartan in the daytime! Eat only substance food. This way you have a reserve in your "bank."

Tip #2: *Always eat something just before* going out—a glass of tomato juice, some fresh strawberries, a small salad of sliced tomatoes and carrots. The point is to get something in your stomach before you go out. This way, when the sight of food and food smells hit you, you will be forearmed! If your stomach is "rumbling" when you arrive you are liable to attack the first sign of an hors d'oeuvre.

Tip: Drink water—tons of it! A large glass of water is a reviver, it is healthful (helps clean the body of toxins) and it is filling! Add a slice of lemon or lime or a sprig of fresh mint.

• Make your meals look attractive . . . a pretty napkin, a lovely china plate, a flower nearby!

• **Eat slowly!** Do not read or watch TV while eating — it's too distracting. Concentrate on the act of eating slowly. You will be surprised how filled and satisfied you will feel.

Trick: In the middle of your meal get up and walk around if you can. This helps prolong the eating ritual. Also the break helps take the focus off that "starving person in front of first meal in days" feeling.

Trick: If you work or are on the go all day: *Pack a snack bag.* A plastic bag of carrot and celery sticks, one or two small cans of tomato juice (the individual serving kind with the zip-open top). When your energy flags the tomato juice is a great low-calorie reviver (potassium)! The celery and carrots do the trick when you need to munch.

Trick: When you get a midday food craving, exercise!

1. A few minutes of aerobic exercises get your heart and blood going—jumping jacks, jogging in place bringing knees high, a brisk walk, always breathing deeply and rhythmically!

2. Or do detensing exercises *concentrating* on your breathing and on your muscles relaxing! Result: *Gets your mind off your "stomach."*

HOW TO SHOP

Ground Rules

• **Take a hard look in your closet.** If you find things you haven't worn for two or three seasons, take them out. Study them and try them on. If they no longer fit or are out of style, check to see if any easy alteration will make them work again, i.e. slightly narrowing the legs of your favorite gray flannel trousers . . . ½" off the lapel of a great tweed blazer . . . shortening the hem of an ankle-long jersey dress to make it work for restaurant dinners Otherwise, *get rid of them*!

• *Get rid of anything if it no longer (or never did)* fit into your *lifestyle,* for example: Ankle-long cotton peasant skirts if you've moved to a city and *never go* to the country . . . or four long velvet and silk skirts if you rarely wear anything but short evening dinner dresses . . . or that mauve-and-tourquoise-print dress that *you bought because it was on sale,* and it makes you feel as if you're wearing a circus tent! *Study your mistakes.*

• **Determine what you *need* and the priorities of your needs.** A suit or coat for winter is a major investment that takes careful selection. If you need a few new T-shirts to take south and go overboard and buy eight because the colors were irresistible, it is not a major splurge.

• **Do not wait until the last minute to shop** (the day before a dinner party, for example). You risk not finding what you need when you need it. You often have to settle for something not great!

• **Never go shopping when you are depressed!** This is when you do "whim buying" and wind up with expensive mistakes!

• **Know how a store works:** what the *shopping seasons* are, when the best selections are available. Remember that across the country great winter coats appear in August when you're wearing your lightest cotton bare dresses, and that summer clothes are on sale at the end of June when *your* summer is just beginning. **This helps you to take advantage of sales.** Also, knowing what's available and when, you avoid last-minute panic buying which happens when you wait too long to get your winter coat and it's already cold out. At such times, your only choice is to settle for **anything.**

• *Do not be side-tracked by sales racks.* You *may* find the perfect cream jersey dress to get you through those last-minute business dinners or a great pair of white cotton trousers that you *live* in all summer! Or a great bathing suit that you'll need for your winter trip south. But "because the price is irresistible," a velvet coat that's a tiny bit tight is madness.

• **Ask yourself:** "Do you need it?" "Can you *easily fit it into your* life, your wardrobe? your finances?" "*Will it work for you*?" Otherwise, pass! There are no bargains if they don't work for you!

• **Check fashion magazines for guidelines.** It helps to get a sense of what's around, to know that wide trousers are "in." Then, even if you look wrong in them, you won't waste time searching for narrow ones! You will know when there are a lot of good, easy dinner dresses around— and even where to find them— since you *will* need one come September.

• **Call ahead to stores to make sure they have what you're looking for.** It helps to know that the lined raincoat you need won't be in for two more weeks!

• Always ask to *speak to the department buyer* when you feel that salespeople aren't ready with the right answers!

• **Learn to buy in groups.**

Often buying from one designer helps, as a designer collection is put together in such a way that pieces go with other pieces: same fabrics, colors, tones in different, "marriageable" shapes. Not only does this make shopping easier, *but by buying additional pieces, you are building a wardrobe with easily interchangeable looks, from day to evening almost anytime of the year!* If you're looking for a suit and there are trousers to match, BUY THEM! When you buy a gray flannel skirt and you haven't the right shoes and pullover to work with it, try to *find them at the same time.* This prevents the skirt's hanging in your closet because you've nothing that "quite works" with it. Secondly, the realization that you *do* need pieces to go with the skirt helps you decide if the whole "investment" is worth it! Thirdly, if you wait, you take the risk that the store might be out of stock when you *do* need additional pieces! **The point is to avoid useless buying and buy *only* if the pieces will perform in your life.** *Perfect example*: the tweed skirt, trousers and jacket . . . the solid silk blouse that matches perfectly, and a silk skirt that matches the blouse (which also makes a "dress"!), and a bare silk top that matches the skirt (a dinner dress!) That's investment shopping!

• **Learn about fit** (see Alteration Section). Know the difference between too small as in *tight*—as opposed to snug—as in a knit top which is supposed to *hug* your shoulders . . . or the difference between oversized as in *perfectly* loose—

and just plain enormous (you really need size 8 and there are only 10s). *Don't let a salesperson talk you into it!*

• **Buy the best you can afford.** Two cashmere or lambswool pullovers in the colors that *work* in your wardrobe will last four or five seasons and will always *feel* like you're wearing the *best*. **That's an investment** even though the initial purchase is expensive. Six not-so-good wool pullovers in colors or textures you don't like but were a "buy" will wear out quickly. You will never *enjoy* wearing them. *That's the whole point of dressing*! They won't be moveable and easily marriageable in your wardrobe day and evening, season after season.

Shopping Tips

• Buy conservative shapes and tones first. They have the longest life! When you're looking for a coat, look for a tone and shape which will work *with what you already* own! A classic shape is an investment; you will wear it with joy year after year (i.e., a trenchcoat). When you don't own a good raincoat and you're out to find one, don't be tempted by that pale rose rubberized cotton ¾ rain poncho that you saw in some

magazine photograph on a mountain in Peru! It may be fashionable and adorable, but unless you can well afford a near useless splurge, *pass*!

• If a shape works for you, don't be afraid to buy a lot of it. A perfectly proportioned silk blouse "with just the right collar for you" is a find! IN-VEST IN IT. *If it comes in several great colors, buy them.* If you wear a lot of cream blouses, *buy two or three in cream.* (One will always be in the laundry.) This is not gluttony—it is taking advantage of a discovery. You probably won't see another one as good for many seasons! **Key: You must ask yourself: Is it right for you?** Is it *classic* enough so you will wear it and *love* wearing it for seasons? This goes especially for shoes. When you've found a shoe that lasts and is a shape that works for you, buy a pair of brown kid pumps and the *same* in black . . . and even in gold for night . . . This is *smart shopping*. It saves time too! You won't have to search for weeks or be caught short when dinner-partying time comes!

Close-Up

• *Know your needs. Arm yourself with a plan, then buy.*

TIPS ON ALTERATIONS

KEY: Know when to alter and when it is not worth it. Know the difference between "tight" (too small) and "snug" (a fit meant to *hug* the body) and the difference between big (as in too-big, wrong size) and oversized (a fit which is meant to skim the body loosely and softly). It has to do with "feel" and the look of the proportion to the eye! Remember: most anything can be remade—taken apart and put back to accommodate—but this is very expensive and takes a true, expert hand which is very hard to find. We are not talking about "miracle work." We are talking about **the little retouching** that can make all the difference in fit and therefore in the **joy of wearing.** These can be done by most any local tailor or seamstress.

• **Key: ¼″ to ⅛″ can make all the difference!** In a jacket falling at the right or wrong spot, in the correct hang of a skirt, in making you look and feel *perfect* in something and thereby *wearing* it a lot, as opposed to letting it hang forever in the closet! Remember: *Never be talked out of your ⅛″*!

• *Before a fitting*, ask your seamstress: Is there room for change? Is there enough seam allowance? Will the fabric remain marked by old hem or seam? Soft-faced wools such as tweeds usually can be steamed to remove hem creases. Hard-faced wool such as gabardine always risk remaining marked! Silk is tricky; velvet is nearly impossible! Darker colors "mark" less than light ones!

• *Always insist on a second fitting.* (1) Ask to have hems or seams basted so that you can have a *proper* second look. Remember, pins in fabric never allow for the proper line and fall of fabric. (2) Always look at yourself in a *three-way mirror* so you can have the best angles to check alterations without having to twist around to see (thereby changing the shape). (3) *Walk around in the altered garment*. Sit down. Stand up. Feel how it feels; watch how it moves. Does your coat or jacket "puff up" at the bosom when you sit? Does your skirt pull across hips? When you walk, does your hem *feel* like it's hitting your leg in the right place, as opposed to too short or too long? Do your trousers "ride up" in the crotch when you sit or walk?

Do they hit your shoe correctly or do they show too much ankle when you walk? Do they "break" too much on your shoes?

• **Begin at the top.** Collar and shoulders must hang correctly, as clothes fall from them.

• Remember, *always do hems last.* If there is taking in or letting out to do on a garment, have it done and *completed* and pressed! Only then have hems measured. The difference in the "hang" of a sewn and *pressed* garment and the "hang" of a basted and unpressed garment is vast. *Always wait to do hems!*

• *Collars:* There is an adjustment needed if: (1) You feel your collar "pushing" against your neck or *looking* as if it's riding up your neck. Keep the second vertebra as a median

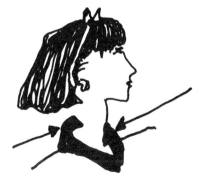

for where a balanced collar should sit. (2) A collar sits back too low and you feel a push at the front of your neck. These tricky adjustments mean rebalancing the entire garment.

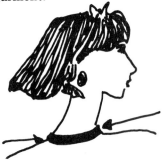

• Make sure the curve of a collar is an "even" curve—that it does not curve up too abruptly at sides as round or cardigan necklines sometimes do. The point is balance and a *flattering* line of curve. *Keep collarbone as a median* for where the curve of neckline should graze and the top button of a shirt should begin, at center front.

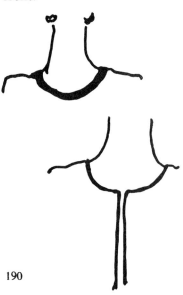

• Remember that you can easily have the points of collars trimmed down and wide lapels narrowed on coats and jackets. This can make all the difference between a "discard" and a "new life" for a favorite blazer. Have the collars basted first to check proportions! Trick to update a shirt with a collarband: Have collar removed and leave collarband.

• ***Shoulders***: Shoulder seams should sit on shoulders squarely and comfortably—no drag or pull, or something is wrong!

• Shoulders should extend between ¼″–½″ from natural shoulder, depending on fabric and whether the garment has shoulder pads or shirring, etc. **Shoulder and armhole alterations are** costly because of the work involved. The sleeve usually has to be removed completely and then rebalanced. This is vital to have done properly because the whole fit, hang, and balance of the garment, dress, jacket, coat, whatever, depend on the shoulder fit. Trick for overly broad shoulders: Moving in the shoulder seam of a jacket or blouse ⅛″–¼″ can give the **illusion** of narrower shoulders!

• For an illusion of width, add a ***touch*** of padding. This can also be very helpful to correct the "fall" of a silky, thin crepe, or thin jersey jacket or top. A tiny bit of padding can help smooth the shoulder line into a neat horizontal and keep the garment from "collapsing"— thereby sharpening and elongating the entire line!

• Be careful about *removing shoulder pads*. If a garment *is* constructed with pads, *by totally removing them you will be left with an excess of fabric* that has nowhere to go but to "deflate." Always leave *some* padding (even a little) in and adjust around it!

• ***Sleeves***: Jacket and coat sleeves should cover wristbone or just graze top of hand when bent upwards. Shirt and blouse sleeves should be a bit longer: to the point where thumb begins to curve out from wrist. This way a tiny bit of shirt always shows below jacket or coat, a pretty and enriching touch. Nothing looks skimpier than shirt-sleeves which are too short . . . as if one has outgrown them!

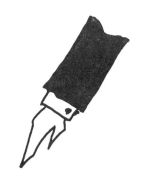

• **Bust**: The rule: *never bust darts on anything*! And remember you can't remove them from garments! Careful fitting of side seams and artful steaming of fabrics should eliminate any need for them.

• **Waist**: Wide waistbands are bosom emphasizers, hip emphasizers, and leg shorteners. They give the illusion of *a lot* of waist. They draw the eye to that area. *The more emphasis on length of torso, the shorter one's legs appear*! A 1″ wide waistband is a good median! Waistbands on trousers and certain skirts often need adjusting in back. Everyone's lower back curves differently depending on curve of spine as well as derriere size. Often trousers and skirts meant to *fit flat* across the lower back have waistbands too straight all around for one's overall shape. The result is a pocket of excess fabric between waist and curve of derriere. They need to be lowered center-back to compensate for the curve of the spine. An easy alteration, though expensive, because the entire waistband must be removed and repinned. Make sure the "recurving" is so gradual that you can't see it!

• **Hem Lengths**: The right hem length depends upon (1) your body and (2) what you are wearing! *It is determined by the point where your leg curves, not by heel height.* There is an easy guide: Take the point at the back of your leg just where your *calf curves in* towards the *back of your knee*. If the hem grazes that point where the curve begins you've got the good median. Adjust up or down ⅛″, ¼″, ½″ depending on how long and lean your leg, and how thin and floaty or narrow and heavy the fabric!

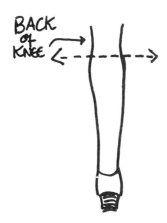

• Here are some rules: The narrower the shape, the heavier the fabric, the darker the color, the closer you keep to calf-curve.

• Remember: a narrow skirt moves up as you walk. Make sure you test the length by walking. If you always keep the back of knee covered, you are keeping a good, balanced length. No one has a pretty back-of-knee or, for that matter, front of knee either! If you have heavy muscular calves or short legs, by *grazing* the curve

so that you just hide the point where the calf curves *in*, you are at the most elongating proportion possible for your legs! The fuller the skirt, the thinner the fabric, the lighter the color, the ¼″–½″ (or more) longer or shorter you can go. Remember, fractions!

• Thin, floaty skirts of silk, chiffon, and cotton gauze can feel and look delicious fluttering around your legs when you walk! Wear them longer (even to mid-calf), especially if they are for late-day! Full, moving skirts can also go a tiny bit shorter than medium, as the "fullness" means movement away from the body. You can often keep a lighter, more airy look by going ¼″–½″ shorter than " median." *It's all in the testing*! Thin, silky pleats of skirts and dresses for day can go ½″–1″ down from median (or even ¼″–½″ up) depending on your height, leg length and shape, weight, etc. Fractions of an inch are still key—too long and it's dowdy, too short and it's dumpy. Always try on skirts with the shoes and stocking tone you will wear to judge the correct proportion.

• **Remember** there is also a point when too-short has the opposite effect! Too much knee "beginning to show" can be a leg-shortener. That is why basting a hem and walking around to check is vital.

TIPS ON ALTERATIONS

• *Remember*: Do not leave too deep a hem turnback. (The child hangover of "She will grow into it!") Too deep a hem will make any garment hang badly: 2″ is more than ample.

TRICK: If there is a mark left after lengthening a skirt or trousers, you can often camouflage it by turning it into a welt-stitched edge. Stitch along mark and then ¼″ below to make welt. Test how it will finally look by having your tailor draw out the lines with chalk to see the final proportion.

TRICK: Often, and especially on chiffon floaty dresses and full, silky ones you find machine-rolled hems (less expensive finish!). You can instantly improve the look and fall of the skirt by having the hem redone by hand. This is expensive as it takes time and patience, but *well worth it* if the skirt or dress (or even pajama) is going to do important evening duty! It instantly looks more expensive and prettier!

• *Trouser hems:* Heel height is key. Always wear the median shoe height (or the exact shoe) which you intend to wear with trousers to do hem. The shoe instep should be covered and the fabric should just **graze the top of the shoe.** When you walk, the trouser should *keep* grazing top of shoe. If you

also intend to wear a *higher* heel than the median, a little "break in fabric" could be added—¼″ should do it! Then you can wear both heel heights!

• *Jacket hems:* Remember, lengthening or shortening a jacket by as little as ⅛″ or ¼″ can make all the difference! A fraction can lift and lengthen the silhouette. It can cover what needs to be covered (the widest point of thigh, very bottom of derriere) by lengthening a "hair." It's definitely worth the time and money! Note: When shortening a jacket, make sure that at least ¾″ remains between bottom of pocket and hem if the jacket has patch pockets of any sort. Otherwise you knock the balance off and it shows that you have done alterations! *The key to alterations is to improve the look of a garment without ever being detected!*

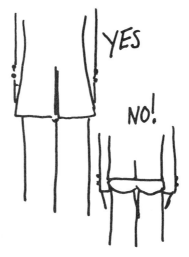

• *Narrowing (or letting out) seams:* Side seams must fall plumb straight along sides of body. Center seams, front and

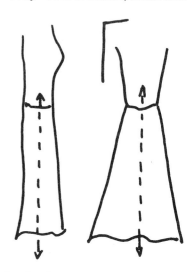

back, the same. This goes for skirts, dresses, coats, jackets, trousers, anything! Never try to save time and money by insisting (or allowing) that a skirt, for instance, be taken in along one seam only. *Taking in or letting out must be done gradually*—the same fractional amount in *each* seam of garment all around! The only time this *doesn't* hold true is when the back—or *front only*—of a garment is too big or too small. You can judge this easily if you watch where side seams rest along body when the excess is gathered in—or where the tight part is, conversely, when let out. *This is why second fittings are vital!* You can only judge this "balance" after the garment is basted.

- Key: Make sure *all* seams lie flat and smooth, never pucker or snake around. Otherwise, redo!

- *Button trick*: the fastest way to *remodel the look of a garment is to change the buttons.* Replace fancy with plain four-hole buttons (or two-hole ones if the button is very small as on a blouse!). Match them to the tone of the garment. It looks more expensive!

- Remember a button should never be sewn flat and tight to a garment. It must have a shank of thread behind to allow space to button freely without pulling the fabric to which it is attached. Have buttons sewn on professionally, especially on "important pieces" such as coats and jackets. They look better (with invisible stitching!) and usually stay on longer since they are sewn with proper thread, etc., *and* never pull the fabric!

Clothes Maintenance

- Always use the best dry cleaners available. Most cleaners cost a fortune anyway and, if you get back a ruined garment, where was the "bargain"?!

- Hang trousers over hangers that have well-padded horizontal bars or clip-hang them from waist, *not cuffs*. This keeps cuffs from getting clip marks. Usually the waistband is covered by a belt or under top so any clip marks are hidden.

- For skirts and trousers: If the fabric tends to mark (velvet, soft wool, etc.), the safest way to hang it is to tuck squares of muslin or tissue between the clips and the fabric!

- Make sure jackets and coats are hung on hangers wide enough to fill the span from shoulder seam to shoulder seam—*not less*, and *not more!* This keeps them hanging straight, with no hanger marks or backs stretched from collapsing on hangers that are too small.

- Make sure dresses, blouses—anything of fragile or thin fabric especially—hang on well-padded hangers that aren't too wide. This avoids marks and stretches along shoulder seams and the horrible surprise of those impossible-to-remove stretch "pockets" in upper sleeves.

- Never hang knits. They will grow! and grow! and grow!

- *Never hang jersey* if it's at all limp and fragile. Like knits it, too, will grow.

- *Never hang anything bias!* The nature of bias is that it will grow and grow forever when left suspended. You risk having totally uneven snake-hems and stretches.

- *Never hang anything with sequins or heavy embroidery.* The weight of the decoration will strain the attached threads and break them and also stretch the base fabric. These garments are best stored flat and folded as little as possible. Always fold them over tissue paper to keep creases and folds from marking the fabric. Store flat on shelves, in drawers, or in boxes at the bottom of your closet.

- **Throw away all wire hangers!** They ruin clothes! Even when paper covered (from cleaners) they tend to eventually mark garments. Always remove garments after being cleaned. To forget often means an unhappy surprise!

- Trick: When closets are particulary crowded, if you slip plastic cleaning bags over garments before "squeezing them in" you can eliminate a lot of creasing!

- For this reason, *plastic bags are a great suitcase packing trick!*

- Remember: *never* store fur in plastic. It keeps fur skins from "breathing" and dries them out!